OXFORD MEDICAL PUBLICATIONS

Immunointervention in Man

Immunointervention in Man

A CRITIQUE OF CLINICAL TRIAL METHODOLOGY

Keith H. Wallace

and

Ronald A. Thompson

Oxford   New York   Tokyo
OXFORD UNIVERSITY PRESS
1991

Oxford University Press, Walton Street, Oxford OX2 6DP

Oxford   New York   Toronto
Delhi   Bombay   Calcutta   Madras   Karachi
Petaling Jaya   Singapore   Hong Kong   Tokyo
Nairobi   Dar es Salaam   Cape Town
Melbourne   Auckland

and associated companies in
Berlin   Ibadan

Oxford is a trade mark of Oxford University Press

Published in the United States
by Oxford University Press, New York

A catalogue record for this book is
available from the British Library

Library of Congress Cataloging in Publication Data
Wallace, Keith H.
Immunointervention in man : a critique of clinical trial
methodology / Keith H. Wallace and Ronald A. Thompson.
p.   cm.—(Oxford medical publications)
Includes bibliographical references and index.
1. Immunotherapy—Evaluation. 2. Clinical immunology.
3. Clinical trials. I. Thompson, Ronald A. II. Title.
III. Series
[DNLM: 1. Adjuvants, Immunologic—therapeutic use. 2. Clinical
Trials—methods. 3. Immune System. 4. Immunotherapy.
5. Monitoring, Physiologic. QW800 W191i]
RM276.W35   1991   615'.37—dc20   91–1955
ISBN 0–19–261918–7 (hbk.)

Set by Footnote Graphics, Warminster, Wilts
Printed and bound in Great Britain by
Biddles Ltd, Guildford and King's Lynn

Preface

Immunointervention is the use of biological products or synthetic pharmacological agents to modify the action of the immune system for the
therapeutic benefit of the patient. The practice is as old as vaccination,
but with the increased understanding of the immune system gained
over the last 30–40 years, immunological therapy is being increasingly
tried as a remedy for many types of illness. These may be either overtly
due to aberrant immunological mechanisms or they may be diseases in
which 'immune enhancement' in some form or other is thought likely to
benefit the patient.

However, an understanding of modern immunology is still not widespread among clinical practitioners or those working in the pharmaceutical industry, and there have been rapid advances in the subject in
the last ten years or so which have made it even more difficult for those
not directly involved to keep abreast of developments. Terms like
'immunomodulator' and 'immunostimulant' have been used rather
loosely and without an appreciation of the underlying processes. This
book endeavours to provide guidance on how to test immunological
therapies in clinical trials and how to critically appraise publications of
such studies. This guidance is set against a background of the general
principles of immunology and its involvement in the disease process.
As will become clear, the immune system does not always operate in
the best interests of the patient.

Chapters 1 and 2 will provide an overview of the basic mechanisms of
the immune system and the ways in which they are involved in disease.
These chapters are not intended as comprehensive texts on these
topics, but aim only to give the reader a general understanding of the
basis for the application of immunotherapeutic agents. Chapter 3
attempts to give some insight into the practical problems of evaluating
the effects of immunotherapeutic agents upon the immune system.
While the clinician is concerned with the clinical outcome of such
treatment, a scientific evaluation should include an assessment of its
effects upon the function of the immune system. This may not always
be possible because the available tests may not provide the most
relevant information. Moreover, the clinical effects of some immunotherapeutic agents may not be explicable in terms of the present
level of understanding of their action or indeed of the immune system

itself, which is extremely complex. Nevertheless, monitoring of immune function should always be considered when designing trials of immunological therapy.

Chapters 5 to 8 comprise a survey of 190 clinical trials of immunotherapeutic agents published in the English language between 1980 and 1989 in four principal therapeutic areas: cancer, infection, autoimmune disease and allergy. A scoring system (described in detail in Chapter 4) has been used to assess critically the quality of design, conduct, and analysis. This has allowed lessons to be drawn for the design of future trials from the attributes and deficiencies of past studies. Brief notes have been included on the proposed mechanism of action of immunological therapies for which efficacy has been demonstrated in trials which achieved a high score ($\geq$ 67 per cent) and were therefore of high quality according to the scoring system. Such a survey is particularly timely because the advent of genetic engineering has recently permitted the generation, in therapeutic quantities, of many immunological mediators, and consequently many clinical trials of such agents are likely to take place in the 1990s.

The importance of the controlled clinical trial was eloquently expressed by Atkins, the President of the Royal College of Surgeons, when addressing the Hastings Centenary meeting of the BMA in 1966. Referring to medical advances such as lime juice for scurvy and penicillin for bacterial infection, he stated: 'Each of these discoveries led to results so striking and so undeniable that no clinical trial was necessary to establish them firmly as therapeutic agents of the first magnitude. Advances in clinical knowledge, however, cannot afford to wait for these rare mutations in human knowledge.' Continuing with reference to some dubious surgical procedures which had been accepted into medical practice without the use of randomized trials, Atkins continued: '. . . the advocacy of a therapeutic measure depends, now, not on the force of personality, the standing in the profession, or the "mellifluidity" of the protagonist, but on more soundly based scientific evidence, and the tool for the forging of this evidence is the controlled clinical trial.' Equally, it would be a great shame if a useful drug, developed at great expense, were rejected because a poorly designed clinical trial failed to detect efficacy.

Atkins' implied themes of the ability of controlled clinical trials to detect small but valuable clinical effects and the avoidance of bias provide the foundation of this book. The finding, set out in detail later, that the published quality of immunological clinical trial methodology has not improved over the last ten years, according to our criteria, provides the justification.

The range of drugs which influence the immune system whether as part of their primary function or as a side-effect is vast and clearly, limits had to be set on the coverage of this book in order to render the task manageable. The following selection rules were therefore applied when deciding whether or not to include a trial in the survey.

First of all, there had to be evidence that the intervention employed some form of immunological mechanism. Secondly, only trials with a clinical rather than immunological primary endpoint were included. For example, trials of prophylactic vaccination were included only if they involved a follow-up survey of the incidence of disease. They were not included if the patients were monitored only in the short term for antibody titres. Hyposensitivity studies in which efficacy was tested by challenging the patients with allergen were included if the route of natural exposure was used. Papers with the term 'phase one' in the title were rejected because the primary endpoints are virtually always tolerance and immunopharmacology. Immunorestoration studies of, for example, colony stimulating factors, were included if there was a clinical endpoint in addition to the recovery of cell counts. Such endpoints included, for example, the incidence of infection or the tolerance of more aggressive chemotherapy. Some studies in which efficacy was assessed by the determination of viral antigen titres rather than clinical symptomatology were included in the section on infectious disease. Thirdly, trials were included in this survey only if they involved at least five patients. Isolated case reports were not surveyed. Finally, there seemed little point in raking over the trials on drugs which have been registered for some considerable time and have become routine therapy. Such agents include Cyclosporin for transplantation, steroids and the NSAIDs for the suppression of inflammation, and the potent immuno-suppressive agents such as Cyclophosphamide. Alpha-interferon was included in the survey, despite its registration for hairy cell leukaemia and Kaposi sarcoma, because it cannot yet be regarded as an established anti-cancer drug for a wide range of cancers in the same way that Cyclosporin has an established role in many types of transplantation. Trials of alpha-interferon in many forms of cancer including some on hairy cell leukaemia and Kaposi sarcoma were surveyed.

The exclusion of trials of Cyclosporin in transplantation meant that this therapeutic area was not included in this survey because the agents currently under development, such as FK506 and Deoxyspergualin, have not yet reached the phase II clinical trial stage at the time of writing. They will be included in future editions of this survey if they undergo human trials. Studies on primary immunodeficiency were not included because the rarity of these conditions, and the ethical

difficulties associated with placebo controlled trials, mean that published reports usually consist of anecdotal case studies rather than
systematic trials.

As will become clear from Chapter 4 the scoring system is not based
on any absolute indicators of quality because no such indicators exist.
The principal aim of the scoring system was therefore to highlight
deficiencies rather than to provide a reliable credibility rating for each
study. All statements have been made in good faith and as objectively
as possible in the interests of enhancing the quality of clinical trials
generally. If the authors have made any errors of fact they of course
apologise in advance. It is also important to make the distinction
between the score assigned to a study and the acceptance of a drug by
the governmental regulatory authorities. Studies which achieved a low
score could be acceptable to the authorities because they will be supplied with a great deal of further information, including the case report
forms and the original protocol, to back up the necessarily summarized
information in the publication. Agents which achieved a high score
according to our criteria may be unacceptable to the regulatory authorities on other grounds such as pharmaceutical formulation, pharmacological, or toxicological data.

Buckingham   K. H. W.
Birmingham   R. A. T.
September 1990

Contents

1

Overview of the immune system

The immune system consists of a number of cells, tissues, and organs loosely arranged throughout the body, but functionally interdependent in a very organized manner. The main functions of the system are the recognition of foreign (non-self) material or substances and their removal from the body. The key element is recognition, with the implication and consequence that a foreign substance previously encountered will, on second and subsequent occasions, engender a more rapid and enhanced response of the immune system, with speedier elimination.

Since the beginning of this century, it has been appreciated that the means whereby the immune system achieved recognition and elimination was by the production of 'antibodies' (large molecular weight globulin proteins). These antibodies are specific for the foreign substance (referred to as the 'antigen'), combining with it to activate the non-specific effector mechanisms of the body (the complement system, phagocytes, etc.), which then promptly destroy and/or remove the antibody-bound substance. A critical feature of the reaction between antigen and antibody is its specificity; i.e., the antibody generated as a result of the introduction of substance A will not react with substance B, and vice versa.

Antibodies are of course produced by cells, so that all the reactions of immunity are ultimately 'cell mediated'. However, antibodies are secreted into the plasma, and their specific immune effects can be transferred to non-immune animals by cell-free plasma; hence this type of immunity is referred to as humoral immunity. For the first half of the century, scientific endeavour focussed on the role of humoral immunity in protection against microbial infection, and this is obviously still an important aspect of the function of the immune system.

However, from the early 30s it became apparent that some types of immune reaction could only be achieved by the presence of living cells, and that the effects could only be transferred to non-immune animals by cells and not by serum. This type of immunity is referred to as cell-mediated immunity. Initially, it was seen to be responsible for delayed type hypersensitivity reactions, but gradually it became clear that this form of immune response was also necessary for defence against facultative intracellular parasites, such as viruses and mycobacteria, that it operated in homograft rejection, and that it was important in defence against cancer—certainly in many forms of experimental tumours.

Cells of the immune system (Fig. 1.1)

Lymphocytes

The lymphocyte—immunocompetent cell   From the work of a number of groups in the 50s and 60s it became clear that the prime cell which initiated the immune response was the lymphocyte, found in the circulation and in most body tissues, as well as in aggregations known as lymphoid follicles, in special widely dispersed organs known as lymph glands (of which the tonsil and appendix are specialized examples) connected by a separate circulatory system, the lymphatic system, and also in two special organs (in mammals), the thymus and spleen (Fig. 1.2). Lymphocytes have a large nucleus and a small rim of cytoplasm.

T and B lymphocytes   Although all lymphocytes are virtually identical under the light microscope, there are two major types, the T or thymus-dependent lymphocyte, and the B, or bone-marrow derived (or bursa-equivalent) lymphocyte. Both cells are derived from primitive stem cells.

B lymphocytes   B lymphocytes make the specific antibody proteins (called immunoglobulins) and differentiate eventually into plasma cells, which are end cells that act as antibody-producing 'factories', the specificity of the antibody they produce being identical to that of the B lymphocyte from which they are derived. They are a minority of the lymphocytes in the peripheral blood (about 10 per cent) and are also found in the bone marrow, in primary follicles in lymph nodes, and in the mantle zone of the white pulp of the spleen, as well as in other lymphoid tissue. B cells are distinguished by specific differentiation antigens on their surface detectable by monoclonal antibodies (CD19, CD20, CD22) and by the presence of surface membrane immunoglobulin. This carries the antigen-binding specificity of the particular line (or clone) of B cells. Once B cells begin to divide and differentiate from primitive stem cells, the antigen specificity of their product develops and becomes fixed, so that eventually 'clones' of cells are formed, each with a different antigen specificity. The process of differentiation and division (or clonal expansion) is antigen driven, but depends on the

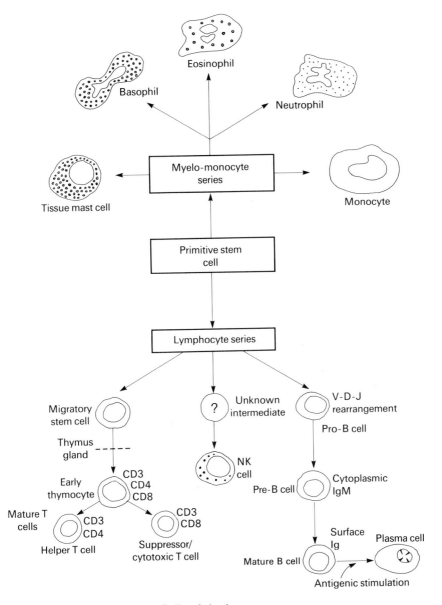

Fig. 1.1 Cells of the immune response.

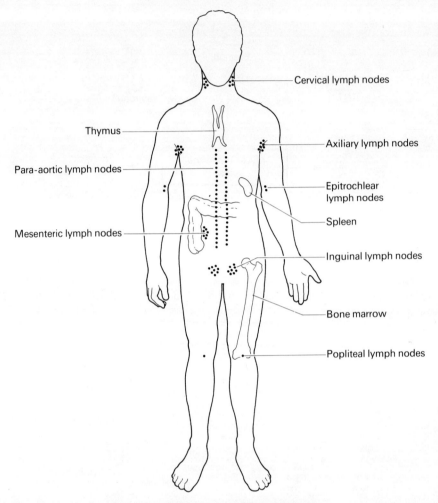

Fig. 1.2 The lymphatic system in man.

co-operation of other cells, notably T lymphocytes and macrophages. In birds (but not in mammals) B lymphocyte precursors need to pass through a hind-gut organ called the Bursa of Fabricius in order to develop the capacity to mature into antibody-producing plasma cells.

T lymphocytes These are also derived from primitive stem cells, but during development they pass through the thymus gland, where under the influence of thymic epithelial cells they develop the antigenic and functional characteristics of mature T cells, before returning to the circulation. This process occurs maximally in foetal and early infant life, when the thymus gland is at its most active, and gradually diminishes during life, so that the thymus becomes atrophic in old age.

T cells are distinguishable by surface antigens recognized by monoclonal antibodies (CD2, CD3) which are a feature of all T cells. Amongst T cells there are two broad groups of cells with separate functions and additional surface antigens (CD4 or CD8). Thus one group of T cells carries the antigens CD2, CD3 and CD4 and the other CD2, CD3 and CD8. T cells are generally referred to as CD4 positive or CD8 positive, the former being the majority of peripheral blood T cells, under normal circumstances, and the ratio being approximately 2:1.

T cells function by recognizing antigens and elaborating small molecular weight polypeptide substances (chemical messengers called 'lymphokines', or more generally 'interleukins' or 'cytokines', since such messengers are also made by other types of cell). These have an effect on cells in their environment, causing the differentiation and maturation of other T cells, and of B cells, and altering the metabolism and enzyme content of macrophages. The means by which T cells recognize antigens has become clearer in the past decade; each cell carries an antigen receptor, or T cell receptor (TCR), elaborated during its maturation and differentiation and carrying the specificity for a particular antigen. This it does in conjunction with the surface molecules called MHC antigens. Once the T cell receptor has been formed, then the progeny of that cell retains the same specificity, to form an antigen-specific clone of T cells. The elaboration and expansion of specific clones of T and B cells is the consequence of antigen administration or entry into the host, and represents the immune response. Some of the T and B cells generated return to the form of small lymphocytes and act as 'memory' cells, able to respond again on future contact with the antigen. These are long lived cells; T cells in particular may live for many years.

Accessory cells of immunity

Monocytes

Principal among the accessory cells are the monocyte–macrophage series of cells. These are phagocytic mononuclear cells formed in the bone marrow, and found in the circulation, in tissues as wandering or fixed macrophages (e.g. alveolar macrophages), as follicular dendritic cells or interdigitating cells in lymph nodes, as 'veiled' cells in lymph, as Kupffer cells in liver, and Langerhans cells in the skin.

Monocytes have a single rounded or notched nucleus with a prominent nucleolus and abundant cytoplasm. The cytosol contains numerous hydrolytic enzymes capable of generating a respiratory burst and killing and degrading foreign organisms. Under the influence of interleukins (especially gamma-interferon and IL2) they become more active and increase their cytotoxic ability.

The surface membrane of monocytes contains receptors for antibodies (FcR) and complement (CR), by which they interact with antibody- and complement-coated organisms prior to ingestion. They perform an important function in the induction of the immune response, in carrying antigen to lymph nodes without completely degrading it, and there interacting with T and B cells, a process known as 'antigen presentation'. They also secrete cytokines, particularly interleukin-1 (IL1), which has a wide range of effects as a pyrogen, initiator of acute phase responses, and activator of T lymphocytes, causing them to synthesize IL2 and express the IL2 receptor.

Monocyte cells are responsible for killing unicellular parasites and some bacterial species such as *Mycobacteria, Salmonella, Brucella*, etc. They do this as a consequence of stimulation by lymphokines, secreted by sensitized lymphocytes. In the absence of the T lymphocyte-derived activation signal, these organisms can live inside macrophages, where they are protected from the host's serological responses, and thus institute a state of chronic infection.

Killer/natural killer (K/NK) cells

These are bone marrow-derived lymphocyte-like cells distinguishable from both B and T cells in a number of ways. They lack the main surface markers of either cell type, but have a distinct marker (HNK1) of their own. They may also have CD2 and Fc receptors, and they have many granules in their cytoplasm, which is generally more abundant than that of resting lymphocytes. They represent only 3–6 per cent of the peripheral blood mononuclear cells and their numbers do not increase during an ongoing immune response.

Their function has been studied *in vitro*, where they are recognized by their ability as cytotoxic cells, either against IgG antibody-coated target cells, or certain tumour cell lines. They are thought to act *in vivo* against tumour cells and virus transformed host cells, but their biological significance is uncertain.

Polymorphonuclear granulocytes

These are the most numerous of the white blood cells. They are characterized by a nucleus with two or more lobes, and they have granules in the cytoplasm. The most numerous are the neutrophils, with poorly staining granules, whose main function is the phagocytosis and removal of tissue debris, foreign matter, bacteria, antibody–antigen complexes, etc.

Eosinophils constitute 1–2 per cent of peripheral blood white cells. They have large, distinctive, brightly staining granules that consist of eosinophil basic protein and heparin. These cells respond to leukotrienes (chemical mediators of inflammation—see below), especially eosinophil chemotactic factor, and migrate to sites of allergic (IgE-mediated) inflammation. Their exocytosed granules modulate the effects of leukotrienes, and the cells are more active and effective than neutrophils in killing roundworms.

The least common of the granulocytes are basophils, with deep blue granules that stain with basic dyes, and consist of histamine and serotonin. The cells carry specialized surface receptors for IgE antibody (Fc epsilon receptors). When IgE antibody is in combination with antigens on the surface of the cells, a series of intracellular events occurs which results in the exocytosis of the granules, causing local smooth muscle vasoconstriction and increased capillary leakage. In addition, the cells synthesize other leukotrienes such as the slow-reacting substance of anaphylaxis (SRSa), eosinophil chemotactic factor, and platelet activating factor, all of which promote inflammation. These responses are a feature of acute allergic reactions. Their counterparts in tissue are mast cells. These are bone marrow derived cells which differentiate outside the marrow. Although containing similar vasoactive amines and mediator systems to basophils, they have an unsegmented nucleus and are widely distributed around small and large blood vessels in the skin, connective tissue, and lungs.

Major histocompatibility complex

The major histocompatibility complex (MHC) is a complex of genes, situated on chromosome 6 in man, which controls the production of cell surface molecules. These molecules are subject to considerable allelic variation within the species, and it is this variation which confers individuality and is important in distinguishing self from non-self. These surface structures participate not only in allograft rejection, but also in immune responses to foreign antigens and in the cytotoxic effects of T lymphocytes.

There are three groups or classes of antigens controlled by the MHC. Class I antigens are the tissue typing surface antigens controlled by three loci, A, B, and C, each with a considerable degree of allelic variation, the alleles being given numbers, A1, A2, B1, B2, etc. These antigens are found on all cells except red blood cells. They are glycoproteins with two polypeptide chains, the larger one carrying the allelomorphic variation, and associated with a smaller 12 kD invariant polypeptide chain, which also occurs free in small amounts in the tissues, plasma, and urine as beta-2-microglobulin. Certain alleles are in so-called 'linkage disequilibrium', that is, they occur together on the same chromosome with unusual frequency, e.g. the alleles A1 and B8 often occur together, and this combination (referred to as a 'haplotype') is associated with an increased frequency in some autoimmune diseases.

Class II or D locus antigens are also controlled by three sub-loci called DP, DQ, and DR, the alleles likewise being given numbers. They are found constitutively on fewer cells and tissues, e.g. in the peripheral blood, they are only found on monocytes and B lymphocytes. However, their expression can be enhanced by interleukins, especially IL2 and gamma-interferon, and they are expressed on activated T lymphocytes and sometimes on tissue cells which are the site of active inflammation.

Class II antigens are associated with immune responses and antigen presentation is class II restricted, i.e. it is only effective between cells sharing the same class II antigens. These surface molecules consist of two polypeptide chains, alpha and beta, each of which consists of a constant region, with a transmembrane and intracytoplasmic portion, and a more peripheral variable region that confers the allelic specificity. Recent studies of the three-dimensional structure of these molecules show a cleft or groove in this variable region, in which it is thought lies the antigen to be presented to the T cell receptor on T lymphocytes.

The genes controlling class III antigens lie in the MHC between the B and D loci. These genes control the synthesis of the complement components, C2, C4 (C4A and C4B), and factor B of the alternative complement pathway, all of which show allelic variation.

As mentioned earlier, the allelic heterogeneity of the MHC antigens is limited in certain diseases with a variety of well recognized disease associations with particular haplotypes. This means that certain MHC antigens or groups of antigens carry an increased risk of certain diseases, and this is interpreted as implicating the response of the immune system in the pathogenesis of the disease. For instance, the class I antigen B27 occurs in more than 95 per cent of patients with ankylosing spondylitis, being otherwise uncommon in the general population, and the haplotype A1 B8 DR3 is found with increased frequency in many groups of autoimmune diseases. How these effects occur is uncertain, but is the subject of much speculation, based on either exaggerated or reduced (inadequate) responses to the relevant antigens.

Nature of the immune response

The events which occur during the induction of an immune response to an antigen, leading to the proliferation of clones of cells specific for the antigen, have been worked out in experimental animals and *in vitro* tissue culture systems over the past 2 or 3 decades.

In vivo, the first (immunologically productive) contact with antigen is usually by tissue macrophages. Foreign material engulfed by neutrophil polymorphs is usually degraded and does not stimulate an immune response. Macrophages, however, carry the antigen to local lymphoid tissue, where it becomes associated with follicular dendritic cells. It is in the lymph node that the key cellular interactions which lead to immunity occur.

Blood lymphocytes, and T lymphocytes in particular, are constantly entering the lymph nodes, by special vessels (post-capillary venules) at the junctional area between cortex and medulla. They move through the gland and leave again by efferent lymphatics, which are eventually collected up in major lymphatic channels in the central abdomen and thorax and are returned to the blood circulation. This continuous circulation of immunocompetent cells maximizes the opportunity for an antigen to encounter the cell or members of the clone which can react with it, because of the predetermined recognition molecules (surface immunoglobulin on B cells, and T cell receptor on T cells) that it bears.

Macrophages, on interacting with antigen, secrete IL1, which causes T cells (CD4 positive) to become activated, and increases their expression of the IL2 receptor (Fig. 1.3). If the antigen interacts with the T cell receptor, then further activation occurs, the cell secreting a number of cytokines. These are IL2 (which enhances macrophage activity, increases the proliferation of other T lymphocytes, and further increases the expression of the IL2 receptor), and gamma-interferon (which increases the surface expression of HLA-DR). Expansion of the clones is concomitant with secretion of other lymphokines IL3, 4, and 5, which lead to differentiation and development of B cells, and IL6, which causes terminal differentiation of B cells to antibody-producing plasma cells. In all of these reactions the lymphokine produces a 'non-specific' second signal, the first 'specific' signal for cell differentiation and multiplication being the interaction of antigen with its specific surface

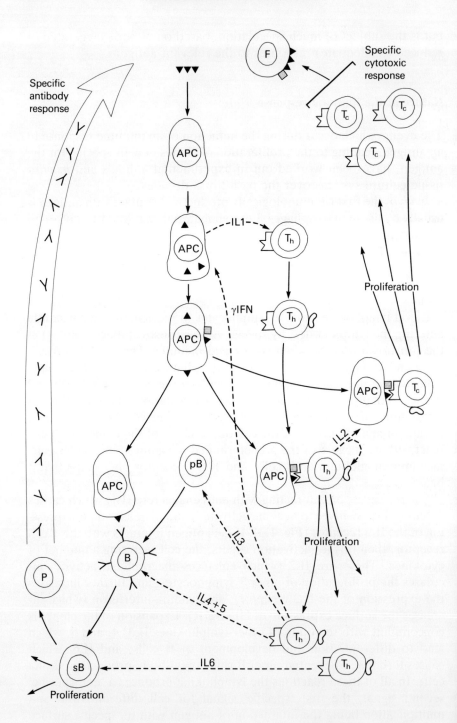

receptor molecules. Thus while there is considerable 'non-specific' cell division and generation of cytokines in a lymph gland at the site of an immune response, only those cells reacting with antigen are driven into the final multiplication and differentiation pathways, leading to the production on the one hand of specific antibody, and on the other to clones of specific antigen-reactive T cells.

Fig. 1.3 A simplified representation of some of the processes involved in the generation of an immune response.

The stimulation of helper T lymphocytes by Interleukin-1 from phagocytic antigen-presenting cells brings about the expression of receptors for Interleukin-2 on the helper T lymphocytes. Subsequent presentation of processed antigen to helper T lymphocytes by the antigen-presenting cells, in association with class II MHC molecules, results in clonal proliferation of the helper T lymphocytes and the release of numerous mediators of cellular division, growth, and differentiation including Interleukins 2 to 6 and gamma-Interferon. Concomitant presentation of processed antigen to B lymphocytes (which does not require MHC molecules) results in the secretion of specific antibodies from an enlarged clone of specific B cell derivatives called Plasma cells. Presentation to cytotoxic T lymphocytes, in the context of class I MHC molecules, results in the expansion of a specific clone of cells which are cytotoxic, by direct cell–cell contact, for target cells bearing the original antigen.

Any diagram such as this can only hint at the complexity of the *in vivo* process which is still far from fully understood. For example, a large number of interactions can be demonstrated for gamma-Interferon and each of the Interleukins, other than the suggested role indicated here. The relative quantitative significance of each interaction *in vivo* is unknown in most cases. There are also other mediators in addition to those shown here. One of the properties of gamma-Interferon which is probably quite important is the induction of MHC molecules on many cell types. This would presumably enhance cell–cell communication (such as the MHC-associated processes indicated above) as well as increasing the susceptibility of target cells to cytotoxic attack. Finally, not all antibody responses require the assistance of helper T lymphocytes. The so-called 'T-independent' antigens, e.g. those with repeating epitopes, such as some carbohydrate antigens, can stimulate B cells directly to produce specific antibodies.

Y antibody; ▼▼▼ antigen; ▲ processed antigen.
Cells:—APC: antigen-presenting cell; B: B lymphocyte; pB: B lymphocyte precursors; sB: stimulated B lymphocytes; F: target ('foreign') cell; P: plasma cell; T_c: cytotoxic T lymphocyte; T_h: helper T lymphocyte. **Cell-surface molecules:**—Y: B lymphocyte receptor for processed antigen (= antibody); ⨏: T lymphocyte receptor for processed antigen; ᘰ: Interleukin-2 receptor; □: Major Histocompatibility Complex (MHC)—class I for T_c and F; class II for T_h. **Soluble mediators:**—IL-1...6: Interleukins 1 to 6; γIFN: gamma-Interferon.

Cells predestined to be specific plasma cells and antigen reactive T cells leave the gland and 'home' to sites where they may encounter antigen (usually in the gut and bronchial associated lymphoid tissue), providing protection against future entry of the antigen.

A single initial contact with antigen produces a response of limited duration and intensity (primary response), while a second and subsequent encounter produces a more intense and longer lasting (secondary) immune response. This is due in part to a switch in the isotype of the antibody formed (from IgM to IgG) in the secondary response, as well as to the stimulation, as immunity develops, of clones with a greater affinity of their antibodies for the antigen, and to an increase in the number of antigen-reactive cells. Hence most immunization procedures to protect against infective disease require two or more injections with the relevant vaccine to confer significant immunity.

Control of the immune response

As with all biological responses, the immune response is under control which limits its magnitude and duration. An excessive response to one antigen would prejudice immune responses to other antigens of biological importance.

Elimination of the antigen is the first mechanism which limits the extent of the response. In the absence of antigen, reactive cells fail to be stimulated and eventually reach a resting phase, so that after a time, the level of circulating antibody and the increased number of memory cells remain as the mechanism of immunity to the antigen. Persistence of antigen leads to persistence of the immune response, and in certain instances to an incomplete switch of IgM antibody production. This occurs in some chronic virus infections, leading to high IgM virus specific antibody as well as high total IgM levels.

The control process is both specific and non-specific, i.e. a process which limits an anti-'A' response must allow an anti-'B' response if that becomes necessary, with the introduction of antigen B. Thus control is initiated *pari passu* with the initiation of specific immune responses. The evidence is that the cells involved in control are T cells functionally and phenotypically different from the T cells which provide 'helper' signals that induce B lymphocytes to undergo differentiation to antibody-producing cells. They are a subset of CD4 positive cells, which operate by inducing proliferation of CD8 positive (suppressor/cytotoxic) cells that effect antigen specific and antigen non-specific control, by reversing the effects of the helper cells.

Another mechanism, first proposed by Jerne, was that of the idiotype anti-idiotype network of antibodies. This arises because when an antibody interacts with a foreign antigen it binds to a surface structural configuration of that antigen, referred to as an 'epitope', by means of a complementary structure or shape in its antigen-binding region (the principle of the 'lock and key'). This structure on the antibody molecule, while technically 'self', is actually a unique structure within the body, and is called the idiotype of that antibody. This generates an immune response, giving rise to another antibody (anti-antibody or anti-idiotype) that combines with it. This anti-idiotype in its binding site has a *complementary* structure to the original antibody combining site, and hence may have a similarity of structure to the antigen. This anti-idiotype can then give rise to anti-anti-idiotypes and so on, the total effect being a balance of positive signals of antigen–antibody (with idiotype), and negative ones due to idiotype–anti-idiotype interactions, limiting the overall extent of antibody production. Anti-idiotype can bind with cell-bound antigen receptor molecules (bearing the idiotype) and limit their proliferation and further differentiation.

Tolerance

This was first described as a phenomenon observed during experimental immunization, but is probably a special manifestation of normal immunological control. It is a specific non-responsiveness to an antigen, and occurs experimentally when the antigen is administered under special circumstances.

It was first described in transplantation when newborn mice of a particular strain were given spleen cells from another (second) strain. They were subsequently able to 'tolerate' skin grafts from the second strain without rejecting them, although rejecting grafts from a third (unrelated) strain of mice. Thus the tolerance which was induced was specific, and was achieved by contact with the cells at a time (in the neonate) of immunological immaturity.

In humoral responses specific tolerance to protein antigens was first observed when the protein was given in its native (undenatured) form in relatively large amounts directly intravenously, rather than by the conventional subcutaneous route. After this procedure the animal failed to make antibodies to the antigen, and subsequent conventional immunization with the antigen produced no immune response. This type of tolerance is of limited duration, but can be maintained by repeated i.v. injections of the antigen. This tolerance is likewise easier to achieve, with smaller quantities of antigen, if administered to new-born animals, or animals *in utero*. There is also a form of tolerance, of shorter duration, which is achieved by the prior administration of very small quantities of antigen (low zone tolerance).

Existing tolerance is broken by giving the antigen in a denatured form, by giving it with an adjuvant, or by giving a structurally related, cross-reactive antigen.

Tolerance is the basis of non-reactivity with self. This is a problem which has puzzled immunologists since the time of Ehrlich. How do the body's immunocompetent cells fail to generate immune responses against self-antigens? McFarlane Burnet proposed the theory of clonal elimination: clones of self-reactive cells encountered self-antigens early in foetal life and were eliminated as a consequence. However, much evidence has accumulated over the years both for and against this idea. In experimental tolerance it is clear that the antigen-reactive cells are not eliminated, but can become active again with the passage of time, or on the institution of a procedure to 'break' the tolerance. Similarly, both clinical and experimental evidence indicates that lymphocytes capable of reacting with self antigens are present in peripheral blood.

Thus the basis of both induced tolerance and natural self-tolerance is thought largely to be because of active suppression of specific immune responses. In patients with autoimmune reactions and autoimmune diseases, there is often evidence of a decrease in the suppressor/cytotoxic subset (CD8 positive) of T lymphocytes, and decreased function of suppressor cells in the peripheral blood. However, recent work from Owen's group on thymic development lends support to the idea that some self-reactive immunocompetent cells are eliminated during thymic development.

The exposure of immunocompetent cells to self-antigens in foetal life at a time of relative immaturity of the immune system would also facilitate the development of natural self-tolerance. Self antigens which subsequently become 'secluded' from contact with the immune system, such as those of the lens, which is relatively avascular, may lose this tolerance. This explains the fact that unilateral trauma to one eye in a child or adult, with exposure of lens antigens to the immune system, may provoke an immune response, and results in subsequent immuno-logically-mediated damage to the other eye—a process called sympathetic ophthalmitis.

Other factors which are conducive to breaking natural self-tolerance and which result in autoimmunity are infections with organisms that may contain self-cross-reacting antigens—referred to as 'antigen mimicry'. This probably occurs in post-streptococcal rheumatic carditis.

There is a strong genetic linkage between certain HLA haplotypes and the development of autoimmune diseases. Consequently, some families appear particularly prone to autoimmune disease, and in others it is rare. This association is strongest with DR antigens, and implies that the possession of certain DR antigens predisposes to the immune reactions that lead to autoimmunity. This may be because these DR antigens are best able to present self-antigens, or are most effective at presenting cross-reactive antigens of specific organisms. Many workers have noted that tissues which are the site of autoimmune disease, such as thyroid epithelial cells, or pancreatic islets of Langerhans —tissues which normally do not express DR antigens on their surface—often express such antigens when they are the site of auto-immune disease processes. This has been taken as evidence that the acquisition of DR expression in a tissue is an early event which sub-sequently leads to the development of autoimmunity. However, it is possible that DR expression is secondary to immune reactions that have already begun, and which represent the initiation of autoimmune processes, since reactive lymphocytes will produce gamma-interferon, which is a potent inducer of DR expression in cells which normally do not do so.

Whatever the mechanism of tolerance, its failure results in auto-immune disease, and ultimately immunotherapy should be aimed at the re-establishment of this specific tolerance.

Antibodies and immunoglobulins

Antibodies are produced by plasma cells, and are large molecular weight proteins with the general name of immunoglobulins. There are five different classes of immunoglobulin (Ig) known as IgG, IgA, IgM, IgD, and IgE (Table 1.1), which differ appreciably in their structure, although having a basic similarity of design. All immunoglobulin molecules have a region with which they interact with their specific antigen, known as the antigen combining site. This is obviously unique to each antibody, and is shared only by immunoglobulin molecules with the same antibody specificity. The pool of plasma immunoglobulins is the product of clones of cells of varying numbers, each with a different antigen binding specificity. Combination with antigen is referred to as the primary function of an antibody. The secondary functions of an antibody are those which are brought into effect usually after antigen combination, namely the ability to activate the complement system, to bind to specific receptors on effector cells, etc. These functions reside

Table 1.1 Immunoglobulins in man

Class	Heavy chain	Mol wt ($\times 10^3$)	Carbohydrate content (per cent)	Mean adult serum level (g/l)	Half-life (days)	Main function
IgG	gamma	146	2–3	12.0	21	Antibacterial Antiviral Antitoxic Main ab in tissues
IgM	mu	970	12	1.2	10	Ab of primary response—mainly intravascular
IgA	alpha	160	7–11	3.0	6	Ab in seromucous secretions
IgD	delta	184	9–14	0.03	3	B lymphocyte surface membrane Ig
IgE	epsilon	188	12	0.00005	2	Anaphylactic antibody

Table 1.2 Secondary functions of immunoglobulins

Immunoglobulin class	Directly opsonizes for phagocytosis (binds to Fc receptors)	Complement fixation		Actively secreted on seromucous surfaces	Reacts with rheumatoid factor	Sensitizes tissue mast cells, basophils	Crosses the placenta
		Classical pathway	Alternative pathway				
IgG	+++**	+++**	+*	–	+++	–	+++
IgA	+ (Fc alpha receptors)	–	+	+++	–	–	–
IgM	–	+++	–	+ (in absence of IgA)	–	–	–
IgD	–	–	–	–	–	–	–
IgE	–	–	±*	±*	–	+++	–

** Subclass IgG1 and IgG3
* In aggregated form (for IgG, subclass IgG2, IgG4)

on the remainder of the immunoglobulin molecule, and they differ
between the major classes of immunoglobulins (Table 1.2).

   The structure of antibody immunoglobulins was initially described by
Porter and Edelmann, and has since been elaborated by many other
workers. The basic unit of all immunoglobulin molecules is a four-
polypeptide chain monomer, with two pairs of chains, one pair of large
or heavy (H) chains and one pair of small or light (L) chains. These
chains are held together by interchain disulphide bridges, as illustrated
in Fig. 1.4. The part of the molecule formed between the light chain and
the adjacent region of the heavy chain is called the 'fragment antigen
binding' or Fab. The rest of the two heavy chains is called the Fc or
'fragment crystalline'. These were first described by Porter when he
treated rabbit IgG with the enzyme papain. Since then, this designation
has been used for all immunoglobulins, all of which are susceptible to
enzymatic cleavage in this manner. The heavy and light chains are
divided into segments or domains of about 110 amino acids each; there
are two domains in each of the light chains and four in each of the
heavy chains. It has become clear that these domains are under the
control of separate genes, for the heavy chain on chromosome 14 in

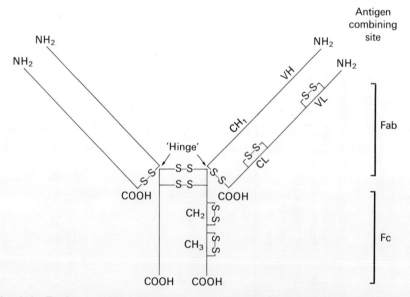

Fig. 1.4   Basic structure of monomer immunoglobulin. Immunoglobulins are
glycoproteins (i.e. carbohydrate moieties are attached to sites on the molecule). The 'hinge' region is the site of enzymatic cleavage of the molecule. VL
and VH: variable domains; —S—S—: disulphide bonds; Fab: fragment antigen binding; CL and CH$_{1...3}$: constant domains; Fc: fragment crystalline.

man, for the kappa light chain on chromosome 2, and for the lambda light chain on chromosome 22.

Variable and constant regions

The domain at the N terminal region of each of the chains is called the 'variable domain', and the others (one on each of the light chains and three on each of the heavy chains) are known as 'constant domains'. The reason for this is that the amino acid structure of the variable domain differs appreciably from one type of antibody to another, and confers the specificity of the antigen-binding site. The constant regions, however, are uniform within the major classes of antibodies, and it is the constant regions of the immunoglobulin heavy chains which carry the sites for the secondary functions of antibodies (i.e. the Fc regions of the molecule).

While there are only two types of light chain (kappa or lambda), there are five different types of heavy chain, gamma, mu, alpha, delta, and epsilon, the names given to the heavy chains of IgG, IgM, IgA, IgD, and IgE, respectively. Thus any IgG molecule will have the peptide chain formula, $\gamma 2\kappa 2$ or $\gamma 2\lambda 2$, and any IgA molecule will have the formula $\alpha 2\kappa 2$ or $\alpha 2\lambda 2$, etc. IgG, IgD and IgE usually only exist in monomeric form. IgM in the serum is almost always pentameric, i.e. made up of five monomer units, each with the formula $\mu 2\kappa 2$ or $\mu 2\lambda 2$, and IgA can exist either as a monomer, or as a dimer. In serum, 90 per cent of the IgA is monomeric and 10 per cent is dimeric, while in external secretions 60–70 per cent of the IgA is dimeric, with a minor portion being monomeric. Polymeric immunoglobulin molecules have an additional polypeptide chain, known as the J chain, which stabilizes the polymeric structure. Dimeric IgA in external secretions has yet another extra polypeptide chain called the secretory component. This is synthesized by the epithelial cells, and there is evidence that it is the means by which dimeric IgA, synthesized by plasma cells in the lamina propria, passes through the epithelium into the secretions. It also confers an added resistance upon the IgA molecule to digestion by proteolytic enzymes, thereby prolonging its action and its effectiveness as a secretory antibody on seromucous surfaces.

Genetic control of immunity—the generation of diversity

Antibodies are synthesized by B cells, which use the genes on chromosome 14 for the heavy chain polypeptides and on chromosomes 2 and 22 for the light chain polypeptides. During differentiation of B cells, the germ line genes are rearranged from their basic configuration to give

DNA segments which can be translated into the immunoglobulin subunits. The junctional regions between the variable and constant heavy chain domains are critical and there are special peptide sequences, coded by genes known as D and J genes, which are shorter than genes coding for domains, but are several in number.

The gene re-arrangement occurs at the stage of differentiation of the primitive 'pro-B cell' to the 'pre-B cell', an immature B cell which expresses cytoplasmic monomer-IgM only, and which occurs in bone marrow and the marginal zones of the white pulp of the spleen. Further B cell differentiation then results in the disappearance of cytoplasmic IgM and the appearance of surface IgM, also in monomeric form. On stimulation by antigen (with appropriate help from antigen presenting cells and helper T cells), B cell differentiation results in the synthesis, glycosylation, and secretion of polymeric IgM, with the additional J chain polypeptide (not encoded by the J genes referred to above) that characterizes polymeric immunoglobulins.

The germ-line contains a finite number of V (V_1–V_n) genes arranged in sequences from the 3' end of the chromosome, and during initial differentiation these are randomly spliced to become adjacent to a particular D gene segment, and then to a J gene segment, so that any individual cell will have as its variable region a VnDnJn segment composed of randomly selected genes. The V and the D gene products contribute to the functional antigen binding site, and hence, assisted by somatic mutation (see below), give the necessary degree of heterogeneity to this region of the molecule to produce the different antigen binding specificities of different clones of cells (Fig. 1.5).

The VDJ segment is then aligned with the constant region genes, the first of which at the 3' end of the chromosome is the μ-chain gene, to give the VDJM of the IgM heavy chain (Fig. 1.5). Similar rearrangement of the VDJK or L segments of the light chains occurs at the same time.

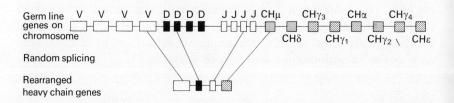

V = Variable domain genes
CH = Constant heavy chain genes

Fig. 1.5 Immunoglobulin gene re-arrangement (heavy chain).

These are expressed in the cytoplasm of pre-B cells as monomeric IgM. Further differentiation leads to the surface expression of monomeric IgM (sIgM) and additional splicing of the delta chain gene to form IgD, also expressed on the cell surface (sIgD). Initially, B lymphocytes express sIgD in association with sIgM, but subsequently, the cells express one or the other, usually with a preponderance of sIgM positive cells.

Antigen driven differentiation leads to further splicing of heavy chain genes according to their order along the chromosome (Fig. 1.5) and to isotype 'switching' (i.e. substitution of the μ-chain gene by other heavy chain constant region genes to give IgG, IgA and IgE). This appears to be modulated by the cytokines IL4 and IL5, with IL6 causing the terminal differentiation of committed B cells to plasma cells.

It follows that once a cell has rearranged its VDJ genes, it has a fixed (committed) antigen-binding specificity, although subsequent isotype switching will determine whether the clone secretes IgM, IgD, IgG, IgA, or IgE. Although VDJ gene rearrangement is random and hence allows an almost infinite number of combinations of different V, D and J region genes to produce a very large number of different antigen binding sites, there is probably a limit to the randomness of the process. Evidence from mice suggests that groups of V genes are used preferentially during normal development, although presumably the potential for a more random utilization exists. Moreover, during the many cell divisions that occur during the process of clonal expansion from the original committed B cells, further random point 'somatic' mutations in the hypervariable part of the V gene occur, to confer the potential for additional variation in the specificity of the antigen binding site.

T-cell antigen receptor

The T-cell receptor (TCR) confers similar antigen binding specificity on T cells. It consists of a disulphide linked heterodimer with extracellular, transmembrane, and intracytoplasmic portions, expressed on the T-cell surface in association with a complex of polypeptides called CD3. Like the immunoglobulin molecule, the TCR has a variable region at the N terminal end of each chain, both together forming the T cell antigen combining site. There are two types of TCR in man, one with an alpha chain and beta chain, i.e. an alpha–beta heterodimer, and the other with a delta chain and gamma chain, i.e. a gamma–delta heterodimer. (Incidentally, these are not the same as the immunoglobulin heavy chains with the same name.) There is no evidence of cross association to form alpha–delta or gamma–beta receptors. The cells bearing the alpha–beta receptors form 80–90 per cent of circulating T cells and the significance of the difference in types of receptor is not clear. Gamma–delta T cells are said to occur with increased frequency amongst the lymphoid cells in the intestinal lamina propria and have been reported with increased frequency in some disease states. Double staining has shown that among gamma–delta positive T cells, there are very few CD4 positive cells, the majority being CD4– CD8–, with about a third CD4– CD8+.

The assembly of the TCR occurs from a similar rearrangement of germ-line V genes, with the random association of shorter D and J gene segments and then splicing to the constant region genes. The TCR is expressed first in the cytoplasm of developing T cells in the thymus, and then on the cell surface together with the CD3 complex of polypeptides. Cells with the alpha–beta TCR express both CD4 and CD8 molecules initially, but then as they develop into mature T cells they lose one or other of the surface molecules before they are released into the circulation, where they populate the T cell regions of the secondary lymphoid organs (e.g. lymph nodes, spleen etc.).

The number and complexity of V genes contribute to the variation of the antigen binding site of the TCR, and it seems that the range of TCR antigen specificities is broader than that of the immunoglobulin Fab region. During the development of the immune response which occurs with continual or repeated antigenic stimulation, the binding affinity of antibody for antigen increases, while that of the TCR remains unchanged. Thus with time and repeated antigenic stimulation, B cell clones with the highest antibody affinity are selected from among the clones with a range of affinities produced in the initial response.

Monoclonal antibodies

Antibodies produced by all the cells derived from one clone have the same specificity. Kohler and Milstein in 1975 reported on the artificial generation of mouse monoclonal antibodies with defined specificity by producing hybridomas or fused tumour cells between a mutant plasma cell tumour line, and normal antibody producing cells from an immunized mouse. The tumour cell conferred potential immortality on the fused cell, allowing the continued expression of the antibody-producing genes from the normal cell. This procedure has been expanded and exploited for the development on a commercial scale of tailor-made antibodies against a wide variety of substances, including specific antigens on T cells, B cells, tumour cells, etc. While these antibodies have been most widely used up till now for diagnostic purposes, mainly *in vitro*, they have been shown experimentally to modulate the function of immunocompetent cells. Their clinical use has so far been limited by the fact that the antibodies are of mouse origin, and their duration of action in man is usually short and terminated by an anti-mouse immunoglobulin response. They have been used to successfully 'purge' marrow of allo-reactive T cells in bone marrow grafting procedures, or to remove residual leukaemic cells in auto-grafting procedures, in the management of leukaemia.

However, it is technically possible to make a mouse–human hybridoma, with the Fab portion of the antibody product having the desired specificity of mouse monoclonal antibody, and the Fc portion derived from human immunoglobulin heavy chains. The molecule is therefore less immunogenic. It remains to be seen how the development of this type of synthetic antibody will proceed, and whether its clinical potential will be realized.

While passive immunization against infectious diseases with pooled normal immunoglobulin, or hyperimmune immunoglobulin is well established, monoclonal antibodies have a greater potential for the treatment of infectious disease, as well as for modulating unwanted immune responses by anti-idiotype antibodies, and in the treatment of cancer.

Interleukins

It was realized early in the studies of cell-mediated immune reactions that activated lymphocytes secreted small molecular weight polypeptides which interacted with other cells and mediated many of the effects observed during such reactions. These were initially given the generic name of lymphokines, and called after the function with which they could be ascribed when studied *in vitro*. Thus there were macrophage activating factors, lymphotoxins, T and B lymphocyte-stimulating or growth-promoting factors, B cell differentiation factors, osteoclast-activating factors, colony-stimulating factors, etc. Since some of these molecules were also produced by cells other than lymphocytes, they were later called cytokines. More recently, they have been given the generic name of interleukins, which emphasizes their important function as chemical messengers between cells, usually affecting their target cell by interacting with a specific cell surface receptor. This nomenclature has been agreed by a Nomenclature Subcommittee of the International Union of Immunological Societies, which has also assigned numbers to molecules with a defined structure and function (Table 1.3).

Table 1.3 Interleukins

	Source cells	Target effects
IL1	Macrophages NK cells T and B cell lines Fibroblasts	Proliferation and differentiation of B cells Lymphokine release from T cells Increased tissue catabolism Induction of pyrexia, stimulation of acute phase proteins. Growth of thymocytes, fibroblasts etc.
IL2	Activated T lymphocytes	Proliferation and differentiation of B cells Growth and proliferation of T cells Increased expression of IL2 receptor
IL3	Activated T lymphocytes Myelomonocytic cell lines	Growth and differentiation of multi-potential stem cells, as well as pre-B cells and mast cells
IL4	Activated T lymphocytes	Proliferation of B cells
IL5	T lymphocytes	Proliferation of B cells. Differentiation of eosinophils
IL6	T lymphocytes Monocytes Fibroblasts	Growth of plasma cells Increased class I MHC expression Acute phase protein synthesis
Interferon-γ (IFN-γ)	T lymphocytes NK cells	Decreased viral replication in cells Decreased cell growth Increased expression of class II MHC and Fc γ receptor molecules Increased NK cell activity Increased antimicrobial and tumour cell activity of macrophages Enhanced action of lymphotoxin (LT) and tumour necrosis factor (TNF)
Lymphotoxin (LT) (sometimes called TNF β)	Activated T lymphocytes	Kills certain tumours and transformed cells, as well as some normal lymphocytes (similar to TNFα)
Tumour necrosis factor (TNF) (sometimes called TNF α)	Activated macrophages (especially by lipopolysaccharide)	Fever, shock, and neutrophil activation Chronically can produce cachexia Enhances viricidal and microbicidal activity

IL1 is produced mainly by macrophages and has a wide range of functions, some specific to the development of the immune response, others involved in acute phase reactions. IL1 induces fever and the synthesis of acute phase proteins. It also causes activation of T cells by stimulating them to produce IL2. IL2 further activates macrophages and other T cells which also increase their surface expression of the IL2 receptor, thereby maximizing T cell activation. Activated T cells also produce gamma-interferon (not yet given an IL designation) which activates macrophages and NK cells, and causes increased expression of class II HLA antigens. IL3, IL4, IL5, and IL6 are also T cell products which act on B cells to increase their growth and differentiation towards antibody-producing cells. Activated T cells and stimulated macrophages also produce lymphokines with related structures and functions and with the historical name of tumour necrosis factor (TNF), which has not yet been re-assigned as an interleukin. TNF has powerful cell killing activity and is thought to play an important role in infections and other pathological inflammatory processes.

Experimentally, interleukins can modulate the function of cell mediated immune reactions *in vitro*, and in experimental animal models. Many are now available in large quantity in pure form using recombinant DNA technology. Thus therapy with alpha-interferon and IL2 is currently being used to stimulate effector mechanisms of cell-mediated immunity in the treatment of malignancy and of infections where these responses are thought to be defective. Colony-stimulating factor has been used to speed the recovery of marrow in conditions of marrow aplasia and agranulocytosis. Undoubtedly these agents will be used in immunotherapy in the future to enhance immune reactions, by affecting the growth and differentiation of cells of the immune system. Another aspect of immunotherapy will be the use of antagonists (monoclonal antibodies, steric competitors, etc.) to counteract the effect of naturally produced (but possibly excessive) interleukins thought to be responsible for harmful pathological reactions. There are already attempts to limit the pathogenic effects of infection by anti-TNF, and this may find wider application.

Complement

The complement system consists of a group of plasma proteins which collectively form one of the plasma activable systems of the body. That is, the proteins exist in an inactive form, and on a suitable stimulus, become activated, usually by means of a sequence of enzyme cleavages, to generate appropriate biological effects. The best recognized of these systems is the clotting system, the final reaction of which, the cleavage by thrombin of fibrinogen to form the insoluble fibrin polymer which is a clot, represents the culmination of a progressive cascade of enzymatic reactions, each component being the substrate for the activated form of the preceding protein in the sequence, and then itself acting on the next in the sequence. While there are similarities between the complement system and the clotting system, there are important differences. The biological roles of the complement system are multiple, and are brought into effect at many points along the activation cascade. While it has been known since the first decade of this century as the system which effected the lysis of antibody-coated red cells, being triggered by the antigen–antibody complex on the surface of the cell, lysis is only one of its functions and is biologically probably of minor importance. Nevertheless, much is known of the sequence of reactions of the system from studies of red cell lysis, for which nine main components, numbered C1 through to C9, are necessary.

The most important biological effects of the complement system are consequent on the activation of the third component, C3, which is the most abundant of the complement proteins. Activation of complement results in attachment of the activated components to the initiating agent (e.g. antibody–antigen complexes) so that they become physically fixed as well as 'fixed' in the sense that they are no longer available for participation in cell lysis. This is the basis of the complement fixation test, to detect antigen–antibody complexes.

There are two major enzyme systems which can bring about C3 fixation, each using a separate set of proteins to generate a specific enzyme, a C3 convertase, which cleaves C3 into two fragments, C3a, a minor peptide with anaphylotoxic activity, and C3b, a major fragment which binds to the cell membrane (or initiating antigen–antibody complex) and mediates most of the other functions of the system.

The two convertases are those of the classical pathway (so called because it was the first to be described) and the alternative pathway. The classical pathway is activated by antigen–antibody complexes, and is much more efficient. The antibodies that do this are of the IgM and IgG1 and IgG3 subclasses, and they activate the first component C1, a multi-molecular complex of proteins C1q, C1r, and C1s, held together by Ca^{++}. C1q forms the attachment to the CH3 domain of the antibody, and activates C1r, which in turn activates C1s by cleavage of a small peptide (Fig. 1.6). Activated C1s then cleaves C4 and C2 in the presence of Mg^{++} to form a bimolecular enzyme, C4b2a, which is the classical

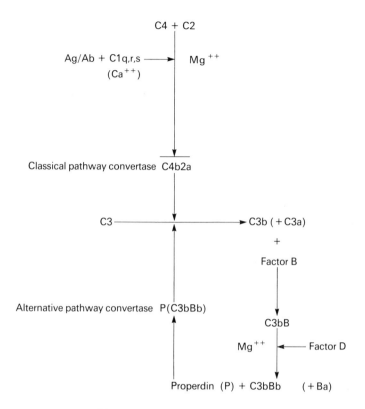

Fig. 1.6 C3 convertases of the complement system.

pathway C3 convertase, able to cleave C3. The reactions are localized to the site of antigen/antibody combination, not only by the physical binding of C1q to the Fc portion of antibody, but also by the fact that cleavage of both C4 and C3 releases a labile thioester bond in C4b and C3b, respectively. This is transiently able to form a covalent ester or amide linkage, which it does to the proteins of the cell membrane or indeed to the proteins of the initiating complex, and the components subsequently remain bound. If this linkage is not formed, the bond is hydrolysed and the component is released into the supernatent as free inactivated C4b or C3b, where its biological role is terminated as it becomes broken down by the specific enzyme inhibitor, known as Factor I. The major inhibitor of the classical pathway, which modulates its action, is the alpha-2-neuraminoglycoprotein called C1 esterase inhibitor. This is a member of the serpin family of proteins, and co-valently binds to activated C1s to inactivate it.

The alternative pathway acts largely as an amplification loop for C3 fixation, however this is generated (Fig. 1.6). It utilizes activated C3, i.e. C3b itself, which combines with a separate protein, Factor B, to form a C3bB complex, which is acted upon by Factor D, an enzyme that in the presence of Mg^{++} cleaves Factor B to Bb and Ba. Bb remains attached to C3b to form the C3 convertase of the alternative pathway, C3bBb, which can then cleave more C3 in a positive feedback loop. This reaction is modulated by properdin (Factor P) and the two proteins Factors H and I. Properdin stabilizes the C3bBb complex and encourages C3 fixation. Factor I, with Factor H acting as an essential cofactor, cleaves C3b and displaces Bb, thereby terminating the reaction. The initial cleavage of C3b is followed by further fragmentation of C3 with release of fragments C3c, C3dg, C3e, and C3f.

The alternative pathway is best directly activated by certain bacterial polysaccharide and lipopolysaccharide structures, and some antibody/antigen complexes, which offer a surface inimical to the action of Factors H and I, thus allowing the unopposed action of the relatively inefficient initial C3 convertase formed between native C3 and Factor B. IgA, IgG2, and IgG4, which do not activate the classical pathway, have been shown to initiate the alternative pathway when present in aggregated form. Alternative pathway activation is relatively inefficient, but represents an important means of eliminating certain bacteria and some virally infected cells in the absence of antibody.

Activation of C3b may also bring about activation of the terminal components of the system C5, C6, C7, C8, and C9, which are known as the 'attack' or 'lytic' components, of complement, and are responsible for cell lysis. C3b itself does not contribute to the membrane damage. The C5–9 components become bound together as a macromolecular complex that inserts into the lipid bilayer of the cell, forming a transmembrane channel that allows the escape of intracellular electrolytes and the entry of extracellular water. This is drawn in by the cytoplasmic colloid osmotic pressure, and the cell bursts by osmotic lysis.

One of the important biological functions of C3 is the opsonization of antibody-coated antigens (or cells) for phagocytosis, since many phagocytic cells, especially polymorphonuclear leucocytes and cells of the monocyte/macrophage series, have receptors for C3b, known as the complement receptor 1, or CR1, as well as receptors for C3b after its first cleavage (C3bi), known as the third complement receptor, or CR3. CR1 and CR3 together mediate the immune adherence and opsonization which result in the elimination of micro-organisms.

The main biological functions of complement are opsonization and the generation of inflammation (Table 1.4). It is also important in man

Table 1.4 Biological functions of complement

Function	Mechanisms	Component
Inflammation	Release of peptides with chemotactic and anaphylactic activity	C3a, C5a, C$\overline{567}$
Opsonization	Coats particles with activated components that interact with specific receptors on phagocytic cells	C3b, C3bi, C4b
Cell killing	Assembles membrane attack protein complex on cell surface —causes functional holes in membranes (trans-membrane channels)	C5, C6, C7, C8, C9 (C5 activated by C3b and either convertase)
Immune complex clearance	C3b coated complexes bind to CR1 on erythrocytes—removed by RE system	C1, C2, C3, C4
	Inhibits precipitation of immune complexes Encourages solubilization of preformed complexes	Classical and alternative pathway
Inhibition of viral activity	Enhances antibody dependent viral inhibition	C1, C4
	Lyses some virally infected cells	Alternative pathway and membrane attack components
Enhances specific immune responses	Interacts with CR2 receptors on B lymphocytes	C3d
	Activates B lymphocytes	C3a, C3b

in immune complex clearance, since human erythrocytes have significant quantities of CR1 which binds the complex through C3b. The erythrocyte membrane protein acts as a cofactor for Factor I cleavage of C3b and subsequent clearance of immune-complexes by the reticuloendothelial system, performing a similar role to the serum protein Factor H, which it resembles structurally.

A few drugs have been developed which modify the action of the complement system by inhibiting certain enzyme stages, but they have proved too toxic for clinical use. Nevertheless, others may be developed in the future, that could limit the degree of complement-mediated

tissue damage that occurs in some auto-immune and chronic inflammatory diseases, and thus become potentially useful in clinical practice.

Inflammation

Inflammation is the natural consequence of infection, trauma, and
chronic antigenic stimulation by intrinsic or extrinsic antigens. It is a
necessary prelude to recovery from infection and subsequent repair. It
involves the liberation of cell damaging factors from host tissue which
act both to attract the host effector killer cells (polymorphonuclear
leucocytes, monocytes, NK cells, etc.), as well as the reparative cells
(macrophages, fibroblasts, etc.), and it provides a cytotoxic environment for foreign micro-organisms.

The process is mediated by low molecular weight peptides which are:
(i) released by proteolytic cleavage during activation of one or more of
the plasma enzyme cascade systems (complement, clotting, fibrinolysis,
kinin formation, etc.); (ii) released during cell-mediated reactions as
interleukins; (iii) released as preformed enzymes or vasoactive amines
by exocytosis of cytoplasmic granules by polymorphonuclear leucocytes; (iv) synthesized by activated polymorphonuclear cells via the
cyclo-oxygenase-mediated metabolism of arachidonic acid to form
prostaglandins; or (v) synthesized by the same cells, as leukotrienes,
via the lipo-oxygenase metabolic pathway of arachidonic acid.

These substances promote chemotaxis, have an effect on phagocytosis, and the killing activity of polymorphs and macrophages, and
also have marked local and systemic effects on the circulation. They
cause smooth muscle contraction as well as relaxation, and increase
capillary permeability. They also affect the interaction of immunocompetent lymphocytes in both a positive and negative direction.

The complement mediators and lymphokines have already been discussed, and the main leukotrienes, prostaglandins and released
mediators are summarized in Table 1.5.

Leukotriene formation and vasoactive amine release occurs as a
consequence of mast cell activation, either from specific allergen-IgE
reactions at surface receptors, or by C5a activation, or sometimes by
other non-specific mechanisms, such as trauma, cold injury, etc. and
even possibly as a result of a very low threshold of reactivity of mast
cells (so-called idiopathic urticaria/angioedema syndromes).

The clinical consequences are those associated with allergic reactions, i.e. rhinitis, asthma, urticaria, angioedema, etc. Many anti-
inflammatory drugs, which form the basis of much of the therapy of

Table 1.5 Inflammatory mediators

Derived from arachidonic acid metabolism		Directly released from cells
Cyclo-oxygenase pathway	Lipo-oxygenase pathway	Platelet activating factor
		Histamine
		Serotonin
Prostaglandin E2	Leukotriene A4	Heparin
Prostaglandin F2α	Leukotriene C4	Proteoglycans
Prostaglandin D2	Leukotriene D4	Kinins
Prostacyclin	Leukotriene E4	Eosinophil chemotactic factor
Thromboxane A2		Eosinophil derived toxic proteins

allergic and related conditions, counter the pharmacological actions of these mediators. In particular, most non-steroidal anti-inflammatory agents block prostaglandin formation via the cyclo-oxygenase metabolism of arachidonic acid. This may paradoxically lead to increased lipo-oxygenase metabolism, with the untoward effects of asthma or rhinitis due to excess leukotriene formation in susceptible subjects.

In the future, therapeutic agents aimed at controlling inflammation are likely to be more selectively targetted at the main types of mediator involved.

Suggested reading

Allison, J. P. and Lanier, L. L. (1987). Structure, function and serology of the T-cell antigen receptor complex. *Annual Review of Immunology,* **5**, 503–40.

von Boehmer, H. (1988). The developmental biology of T lymphocytes. *Annual Review of Immunology* **6**, 309–26.

Crumpton, M. J. (ed.) (1987). HLA in medicine. *British Medical Bulletin,* Vol. 43, No. 1. Churchill Livingstone, Edinburgh.

Jelinek, D. E. and Lipsky, P. E. (1987). Regulation of human B lymphocyte activation, proliferation and differentiation. *Advances in Immunology,* **40**, 1–59.

Kaplan, J. (1986). N. K. cells lineage and target specificity: a unifying concept. *Immunology Today,* **7**, 10–13.

Kindt, T. J. and Capra, J. D. (1984). *The antibody enigma.* Plenum Press, New York.

Klein, J. (1990). *Immunology.* Blackwell Scientific Publications, Oxford.

Male, D., Champion, B., and Cooke A. (1987). *Advanced immunology.* Gower Medical Publishing, London.

Poste, G. and Crooke, S. T. (ed.) (1988). *Cellular and molecular aspects of inflammation*. Plenum Press, New York.

Roitt, I. M. (1984). *Essential immunology,* (5th edn). Blackwell Scientific Publications, Oxford.

Ross, G. D. (ed.) (1986). *Immunobiology of the complement system. An introduction for research and clinical medicine.* Academic Press, Orlando.

Stites, D. P., Stobo, J. D., Fudenberg, H. H., and Wells J. V. (1984). *Basic and clinical immunology,* (5th edn). Lange Medical Publications, Los Altos, California.

Weiss, L. and Greep, R. G. (1977). *Histology,* (4th edn). McGraw Hill, New York.

2

Immunology and disease—an overview of immunotherapy

The unravelling of the mechanisms of the immune system over the past few decades has resulted in a greater appreciation of its involvement in disease processes. Indeed, the processes of clinical observation have frequently stimulated fundamental research into immunological mechanisms, as well as providing complementary information to validate and extend experimental data on the nature of immunity. To give but a few examples, a large part of what is known of antibody structure derived from the study of human myeloma proteins, and the subsequent animal models of myelomatosis. Immunodeficiency states have provided answers as well as questions about the development of the immune system, and organ transplantation and autoimmunity are clinical conditions which have spawned a vast amount of research into the nature of immunological tolerance and other phenomena of immunity.

The immune system can be shown to be involved in many disease states, with the generation of specific antibodies or antigen reactive cells. In some instances this involvement is presumed, based on the histological appearances of lymphoid infiltration of lesions, changes in serum immunoglobulin levels, evidence of complement consumption, or changes in other parameters of immunological activity, without knowledge of the precise stimuli, or of the exact paths by which immune mechanisms are being activated.

In infective conditions, the action of the immune system is usually evident, appropriate, and designed to eliminate the infection. However, it is now appreciated that in some instances this activity may have, *pari passu*, harmful consequences to the host, with destruction of host cells and tissues. Occasionally, the damage to the host produced by the action of the immune system reacting to the foreign micro-organism is greater than that produced by the agent itself. Moreover, a greater understanding has been reached of how different organisms can evade the mechanisms of immunity and survive in the host. This understanding of the various parasite–host relationships has allowed the development of better strategies for parasite elimination. Severe dysfunction of the immune system, either genetic or acquired, leads to the various syndromes of immunodeficiency, or defects in dealing with infections.

In allo-immune conditions, (e.g. organ transplantation, transfusion reactions, Rhesus haemolytic disease of the newborn, etc.) disease is the natural consequence of the action of the immune system, against foreign antigens gaining entry to the host, and attempts have been made to control and suppress these natural immune reactions. In allergic disease, the clinical state arises from a heightened or inappropriate immune reaction to a natural agent in the environment. Therapy aims at either eliminating contact with the stimulating agent, or modifying by pharmacological means the effects of the inflammatory mediators generated during these reactions, or in certain instances, using specific antigen (allergen) immunotherapy, to modify the nature of the patient's immunological reaction to the environmental agent, so that it becomes less harmful, with a consequent beneficial effect on the disease symptoms.

In autoimmunity, the immune system is primarily 'at fault', acting directly against host cells and antigens as if they were foreign and thereby producing disease. This comes about as a failure of natural tolerance. At present, therapy largely entails the use of drugs either to suppress the inflammation which is a consequence of such immune reactions, or to suppress the immune reactions themselves and diminish the production of autoantibody or the activity of the autoantigen reactive lymphocytes. Unfortunately, this treatment has the inevitable consequence of depressing the immune system generally and rendering the patient more prone to intercurrent infections.

One of the functions of the immune system is the control of neoplastic processes, and there is a deal of clinical and experimental evidence to support this role. Thus the development of cancer is seen as a failure of this function in some manner, and a variety of therapeutic strategies have been aimed at correcting the supposed failure by enhancing immune mechanisms, both against specific tumour antigens, and non-specifically by agents which generally 'enhance' the activity of the immune system. It is an unfortunate paradox that most chemotherapeutic regimens against cancer consist of drugs which damage dividing cells, and thus as a consequence they further depress the immune system, which relies on cell division and differentiation for maximum effect.

Immunodeficiency states

Individuals who are unusually prone to infections by common micro-organisms or who develop infections by opportunistic organisms which are not normally pathogenic, are considered to have clinical immuno-deficiency. This may be due to a defect in any of the range of non-specific and immunologically specific factors which keep invading micro-organisms at bay. The skin and mucous membranes are the most effective of the non-specific barriers against micro-organisms, and their damage (e.g. in burns, or in fibrocystic disease) leads to an increased tendency to infection.

Defects in the immune system which result in immunodeficiency dis-eases are either (i) lymphoid or (ii) non-lymphoid, i.e. occurring in the accessory systems of immunity such as the complement and phagocytic systems. The various types of defects can either be primary, arising from a genetically determined disorder or occurring *de novo* from as yet unknown causes; or secondary, occurring as a consequence of some other disease process, such as infection, malignancy, metabolic, or degenerative disease, which may result in depression of a particular arm of the immune system.

Primary immunodeficiency

These disorders are rare, but are important because of the light they have shed on the functions of the immune system. The main disorders are listed in Table 2.1. Primary disorders of lymphoid immunity are divided into (i) those which are mainly defects of antibody formation and (ii) those which are mainly defects of cell-mediated immunity. This division expresses the clinical consequences of the defect, although in most instances formal testing reveals impaired function in both the humoral and cellular arms of the immune response in almost all of the syndromes of immunodeficiency. Antibody deficiency (hypogammaglo-bulinaemia) is the most common form of primary immunodeficiency.

Therapy

Apart from antibiotics to treat infective episodes, the cornerstone of treatment in patients with immunodeficiency is adequate replacement. For patients with antibody deficiency, concentrated pooled normal human immunoglobulin (almost entirely IgG) is the most appropriate and effective treatment. Intramuscular preparations have been used successfully for this purpose since the 1950s, but in the past 10 years a range of preparations suitable for intravenous use have become avail-able, and clinical trials have demonstrated their efficacy. With these preparations it is possible to achieve much higher serum levels of IgG antibody, and lessen the frequency of infective episodes in some

Table 2.1   Primary immunodeficiency diseases

A. *Diseases due to antibody deficiency*:
    1. X-linked agammaglobulinaemia (hypogammaglobulinaemia)
    2. X-linked hypogammaglobulinaemia, with normal or hyper IgM
    3. Selective IgG deficiency
    4. Selective IgA deficiency
    5. IgG subclass deficiency
    6. Antibody deficiency with normal immunoglobulin levels
    7. Transient antibody deficiency of infancy

B. *Diseases with B and T cell defects*:
    1. Severe combined immunodeficiency (SCID)
        (a) ADA deficiency
        (b) Nucleoside phosphorylase deficiency
        (c) X-linked SCID
        (d) MHC Cl II deficiency ('bare lymphocyte' syndrome)
        (e) X-linked lymphoproliferative disease
    2. Common variable immunodeficiency (acquired
        hypogammaglobulinaemia)

C. *Diseases with associated clinical features*
    1. Wiskott–Aldrich syndrome
    2. Ataxia telangiectasia
    3. 3rd and 4th arch syndromes (di George syndrome)

D. *Diseases with abnormalities of phagocyte function*:
    1. Chronic granulomatous disease
    2. Chediak–Higashi disease
    3. Leucocyte adhesion defect
    4. Hyper-IgE syndrome

E. *Diseases with defects of complement components*:
    1. Recurrent bacterial infections (defects of C1, C3, Factor B)
    2. Recurrent Neisserian infections (defects of C5, C6, C7 or C8)

patients. In addition to prevention of overt infections, it is essential to limit the chronic damage to the sino-pulmonary system that occurs with constant low grade infections, and which may lead to crippling cardio-respiratory failure.

For defects of cell-mediated immunity, both of the lymphoid and granulocyte series, bone marrow transplantation is the most effective therapy. Matched sibling donors are best, but some limited success has been achieved by matched unrelated donor marrow transplantation. As with all marrow transplant procedures, graft versus host disease and its management by immunosuppressive therapy are the main hazards. During the time necessary for the donor to be found and for the procedure to be carried out, patients with severe combined immunodeficiency receive passive pooled normal immunoglobulin and prophylactic Trimethoprim (against pneumocystis infection) until evidence of a functioning marrow is obtained. Without marrow transplantation, replacement immunoglobulin by itself does not usually achieve a significant prolongation of life in SCID patients.

Various attempts have been made to treat immunodeficient patients with immunostimulant drugs, some derived from thymic hormones, but there has been little evidence that these agents add anything to the management of any of these patients.

Cancer

Cancer is the proliferation of an altered form of normal cells which have escaped from the usual controls on growth and differentiation. Tumours are invasive and harmful to the surrounding normal tissue and tend to recur, sometimes at a distance from the original site, a process known as metastatic spread. Cancer is harmful because it disrupts normal physiological processes by a variety of mechanical and biochemical means. Tumours may encircle and obstruct the passage of fluids through tubular structures, or they can infiltrate and disrupt the structure of vital tissues and organs. Obstruction of the blood supply can cause necrosis, whilst other tumours secrete non-physiological levels of hormones which cause metabolic chaos locally or systemically. Cancer can affect any tissue of the body, and the incidence of any particular type varies from country to country. In the UK the four most common types are lung, large bowel, breast, and skin cancers.

The first line of treatment for most neoplastic disease is the surgical removal, if possible, of the cancerous tissue. For disseminated malignancy such as cancers of the blood, lymphoid system and bone marrow, systemic treatment is needed. This is usually in the form of cytotoxic drugs with or without radiotherapy. Surgical removal of solid tumours is often accompanied by radiotherapy or chemotherapy in an attempt to destroy any residual tumour, either locally or at a distance from the original site. Radiotherapy alone is most frequently used in inoperable lung cancers, although it is usually palliative rather than curative. Chemotherapy involves the use of non-specific inhibitors of cell division such as: alkylating agents (e.g. Cyclophosphamide), nitrosoureas (e.g. Lomustine), vinca alkaloids, DNA-intercalating agents (e.g. the anthracyclines) and antimetabolites (e.g. Methotrexate—a folic acid antagonist). These agents inhibit cell division in both healthy and cancerous tissue, leading to immune suppression, loss of hair, nausea, and vomiting. The skill of using these agents lies in finding the 'window of opportunity' in which the differential sensitivity of normal and cancer cells to a particular cocktail of chemotherapeutic agents is as large as possible. Substantial improvement in life expectancy has been achieved for some cancers using these agents.

In principle, cancer cells should appear different from the normal cells from which they are derived and hence should be recognized as such by the immune system. Indeed, there is much experimental evidence that the immune system is involved in defence against cancer (for a review see Brodt 1983 and Siegel 1985), and hence the clinical appearance of neoplastic disease represents a failure of the immune system in this respect.

A range of immunomodulating agents and procedures have been used in an attempt to control neoplastic disease, but in the vast majority of cases without significant success. They are used as an addition to the first line treatments of surgery, radiotherapy, and chemotherapy. They include: vaccines consisting of putative tumour antigens with or without adjuvants; immunostimulating agents or adjuvants such as BCG, Levamisole, thymic hormones, etc; recombinant interleukins (e.g. IL-2 or gamma interferon); lymphokine-activated killer (LAK) cells (i.e. the patient's own lymphocytes stimulated *ex vivo* by lymphokines). Plasmapheresis and apheresis are also employed to remove immune complexes and soluble tumour antigens from the blood. Experimentally, even the most successful of immunological procedures only work if the tumour load is of a limited size, and hence immunotherapy should only be attempted after initial treatment to reduce as far as possible the extent of the malignancy.

Autoimmunity

One of the main stimuli to the study of immunology in the past three decades has been the awareness that disease may be the consequence of an aberrant immune response, directed against self antigens. This was foreseen by Ehrlich at the turn of the century, who put forward the concept of the 'horror autotoxicus', and there is much evidence that this is a reality.

The factors which lead to the development of autoimmune disease are varied, but include familial and genetic factors, in particular those concerned with the genetic control of the immune response, as well as hormonal and environmental factors, including trauma, infections, and drugs. There is a close association between susceptibility to auto-immune disease and certain HLA allotypes, especially among the class II antigens, and aberrant class II antigen expression is often seen on the cells of tissues which are the site of autoimmune disease. Many auto-immune diseases are more common in females, and in experimental animal models of autoimmunity the administration of male sex hormones to females retards the development of the disease process. Some auto-immune diseases are preceded by infection or exacerbated following infections. In a few the relationship is well established, e.g. in rheumatic carditis and streptococcal infection, while in others there is an associa-tion of the disease with high titres of antibodies to a particular organ-ism, implying a recent infection, e.g. in insulin-dependent diabetes mellitus increased antibodies to ECHO virus have been described. Some drugs, such as hydrallazine, penicillamine, methyldopa, etc. can induce states of autoimmunity in some patients. All the contributory factors act to break the tolerance of the individual's immune system to self-antigens.

Classification

Autoimmune disorders are classified broadly as organ specific and non-organ-specific. In the former, a particular organ is the site of the autoimmune process and of the disease. These mainly involve diseases of endocrine organs but also include some renal, haematological, and muscle disorders. In non-organ-specific diseases, the autoimmune pro-cess is directed against widely distributed antigens, e.g. nuclei and mitochondria, and the mechanisms by which the disease occurs and affects the tissues and organs concerned are not always clear, although most non-organ-specific autoimmune diseases are multi-system dis-orders.

This classification is illustrated in Table 2.2.

Clinical features

The clinical consequences of autoimmunity depend on the type of immune response generated, i.e. the antigens against which it is directed and the nature and amount of the antibodies and autoreactive lymphocytes formed. In autoimmune thyroiditis, the thyroid gland may undergo infiltration and hypertrophy without significantly affecting

Table 2.2   Autoimmune diseases

Primarily organ-specific diseases
Autoimmune haemolytic anaemia
Autoimmune thrombocytopoenia
Autoimmune thyroiditis (leading to Hashimoto's disease, Grave's disease
  or primary myxoedema)
Pernicious anaemia
Type I diabetes
Primary Addison's disease
Myasthenia gravis
Pemphigus vulgaris
Bullous pemphigoid

Non-organ-specific diseases
Rheumatoid arthritis
Systemic lupus erythematosus
Chronic active hepatitis
Primary biliary cirrhosis
Wegener's granulomatosus

---

overall thyroid function (Hashimoto's thyroiditis), or it may be stimulated to overactivity as a consequence of antibodies directed against the
TSH receptor on the surface of thyrocytes, which mimic the action of
TSH (producing Grave's disease). Alternatively, the gland may become atrophied due to the cytotoxic action of the immune response,
leading to myxoedema. In most organ-specific diseases, however, the
autoimmune process leads to specific damage and loss of function of the
organ or tissue concerned. This occurs in other autoimmune endocrine
disorders such as adrenalitis, type I diabetes, primary ovarian failure,
etc. In autoimmune haemolytic anaemia and autoimmune thrombocytopoenia, the autoantibodies to the cell surface antigens lead to
damage and sequestration of the cells, while in Goodpasture's syndrome, autoantibodies to the basement membrane antigens of the renal
glomerulus and lung alveoli lead to damage, with nephritis and pulmonary haemorrhage. In myaesthenia gravis, antibodies to acetylcholine receptors impair neuromuscular transmission, causing the
weakness and fatiguability characteristic of the disease.
    In non-organ-specific diseases, the way in which the autoimmune
process results in disease is often unclear. However, the autoantibodies
formed may act as a diagnostic marker of the disease concerned, and in
some instances they can be used to monitor progress of treatment,

although in general in autoimmune diseases, there is only a poor correlation between the level of autoimmune activity detectable in the blood (i.e. autoantibodies or antigen reactive cells) and the clinical state of the patients. Such diseases include rheumatoid arthritis, systemic lupus erythematosus, and many of the so-called connective tissue diseases, as well as chronic active hepatitis and vasculitic disorders. They are characterized by particular patterns of autoantibodies to antigens widely dispersed throughout the body.

Therapy

For autoimmune endocrine disorders, the immunological process is seldom apparent until sufficient damage has occurred to impair the function of the gland, and most patients present with glandular dysfunction. By this time the immune process is all but burnt out, and treatment is largely by pharmacological agents which reduce the function of the gland (in overactivity states) or replacement hormones in states of hypofunction (myxoedema, diabetes, Addison's disease, etc).

Most other autoimmune disorders wax and wane, and are subject to natural remissions and exacerbations. Treatment is mainly aimed at ameliorating the effects of the immunological reactions by anti-inflammatory agents, usually corticosteroids, until a period of natural remission occurs. In severe cases, immunosuppressive therapy to dampen down the aberrant immune response is needed, although it brings the attendant hazards of secondary immunodeficiency. The variable natural course of these disorders makes evaluation of therapy particularly difficult.

Clinical allergy

Aberrant or excessive immunological responses to non-replicating chemical substances can be a cause of much morbidity and indeed mortality. The substances which provoke these (allergenic) responses vary from metals to simple chemicals to pharmacological agents, as well as more complex peptides, polysaccharides, and proteins derived from micro-organisms, plants, and animals. The factors which produce such abnormal immunological responses are varied and peculiar to an individual and his environmental circumstances. They include factors in the individual's genetic control of immune responses (MHC, suppressor cell activity, etc.), as well as the age, duration, and route of exposure to the relevant agent and its nature. Some individuals are particularly prone to allergic reactions such as asthma, hay fever, and eczema, and are referred to as having an allergic or atopic constitution. They are often sensitive to many of the common environmental allergens. Some agents are potent allergens and will induce hypersensitivity states in the majority of the population, if exposure is prolonged sufficiently. Such agents are simple chemicals such as picryl chloride or di-nitro-chlorobenzene, and complex bacterial enzymes or plant extracts if inhaled over a period of time. The respiratory and gastro-intestinal tracts are common routes of sensitization, and most allergic reactions are initiated via these routes early in childhood, when both the non-specific and immunological (IgA-mediated) barriers to macromolecules at seromucous surfaces are least well developed.

Classification

Allergic symptoms depend in part on the nature of the immune response and the type of hypersensitivity that has developed to a particular antigen (allergen). They also obviously depend on the degree of exposure to the relevant allergen (a purely pollen-sensitive individual will be asymptomatic outside the pollen season), and on the level of responsiveness of the individual's effector mechanisms, which are triggered by the particular immunological reaction. Some people who have evidence of IgE-mediated antibodies will nevertheless not experience symptoms at quite a high level of exposure, while others with an equal level of antibody will be prostrate on minimal exposure. The precise nature of the symptoms, i.e. asthma or hay fever, depends on non-specific factors which control antigen entry, as well as the local density of mucosal mast cells which trigger IgE-mediated reactions.

Hypersensitivity reactions have been classified into four types, numbered 1–4. This original classification, first described by Gell and Coombs in 1958, has stood the test of time, and most allergic symptoms are the result of the action of one or more of these hypersensitivity reactions.

Type I is IgE mediated, i.e. individuals who form appreciable amounts of IgE antibodies to environmental allergens are likely to develop such symptoms. It is the commonest form of clinical allergy, and it is reckoned that up to 20 per cent of the population have the tendency in varying degrees to develop this type of sensitivity at some time in their life. The symptoms occur because IgE antibodies are bound to receptors on mast cells, and in the presence of the antigen, cross-linking of surface IgE molecules occurs, and as a result the mast cells discharge their granules consisting of histamine and potent vasoactive amines. They are also stimulated to synthesize other pharmacologically active molecules known as leukotrienes, which together cause local vasodilatation, increased capillary permeability, and smooth muscle contraction. In some individuals, IgG antibodies of a particular subclass can be shown to produce the same effect, but the clinical relevance of these antibodies is uncertain.

Type 2 reactions are produced mainly by complement fixing IgG antibodies, which develop to antigens on the surface of cells. The best characterized of these are antibodies to blood cell surface antigens, which may be intrinsic (i.e. autoantibodies) or adsorbed extrinsic antigens. This is usually the case in pharmacological drug hypersensitivity, where the drug adsorbs to the red cells and the anti-drug antibody reaction (with complement) on the cell surface causes haemolysis and haemolytic anaemia. Similar reactions have been described with drug-induced thrombocytopoenia and granulocytopoenia.

Type 3 reactions are also mainly IgG mediated, and occur when antibody and soluble antigen form complexes in the tissues, or in the circulation. These complexes activate the complement system and generate inflammation (as would an infective agent). In the tissues the result of constant inflammation will produce acute and chronic damage in the sites where the reactions occur. This usually happens with high levels of antibody and constant exposure to the allergen, and is a feature of allergic alveolitis, and some forms of gastro-intestinal food hypersensitivity. Where the antibody level is low and the antigen exposure high, soluble immune complexes may form which enter the circulation and are then deposited widely at end capillaries, producing vasculitic damage in the kidneys, skin, synovia, pleura, and pericardium, and a multi-system clinical picture. This is seen in serum sickness, an illness of fever, joint pains, and nephritis, resulting from the injection of foreign (usually horse) serum, and occurring after 7–10 days as the individual's immune reaction to the foreign proteins develops. It is obviously uncommon now, since the use of heterologous sera in clinical medicine is rare.

Immune complex tissue deposition, sometimes with vasculitis, is a feature of many disorders in which the precise aetiology and often the nature of the antigen or antigens involved is obscure. The antigens may be extrinsic or intrinsic (part of an autoimmune process). Extrinsic antigens are often derived from infecting micro-organisms, and such complexes represent a mechanism by which the immune response to an infection produces pathological damage. In some disorders, such as Henoch–Schoenlein purpura, or dermatitis herpetiformis, or Berger's disease, the complexes are largely of IgA, and the presumption is that the antigen is mainly stimulating the secretory immune system and is situated in or enters via the gut or respiratory tract.

Type 4 reactions occur when antigens interact maximally with antigen sensitized lymphocytes. These produce lymphokines, which result in local inflammation. This is a more slowly developing hypersensitivity, and is characteristic of skin contact sensitizing agents such as metals (especially nickel) and some topical antibiotics, which can produce an allergic dermatitis.

Therapy

Therapy is aimed mainly at allergen avoidance, together with the use of pharmacological drugs (antihistamines, steroids, etc.), which inhibit or counter the inflammatory effects of the immunological reactions.

Immunotherapy is only indicated for IgE-mediated hypersensitivity, and is contra-indicated in other forms of allergy. It can be effective, especially in severe allergic reactions to insect venoms, and in some inhalant allergies. It consists of giving gradually increasing doses of the allergen by subcutaneous injection, starting with minute concentrations, in an attempt to 'divert' the individual's immune response from an IgE to an IgG response. The mechanisms by which the procedure is effective in relieving symptoms are probably complex, and in addition to forming so-called 'blocking' antibodies of the IgG class, involve increased activity of suppressor cells, as well as modulation of the effector mechanism expression.

There is experimental and some clinical evidence that immune complex disorders may arise as a consequence of a degree of immunodeficiency. The immune response occurs, but is not sufficient to completely eliminate or suppress the infection, so that a low grade chronic infection may result, with persistent release of antigens from the micro-organism. These react with antibodies of low affinity to form immune complexes which circulate and are deposited in various tissues to cause the immunopathological state. This concept has resulted in efforts to treat some immune complex diseases with so-called immuno-stimulating agents such as Levamisole and thymic hormone preparations, but with little consistent clinical benefit.

Suggested reading

Brodt, P. (1983). Tumour immunology—three decades in review. *Annual Review of Microbiology,* **37,** 447–76.

Haeney, M. R. and Chapel, H. (1989). *Clinical immunology*, (2nd edn). Blackwell Scientific Publications, Oxford.

Kumar, V., Kono, D. H., Urban, J. L., and Hood, L. (1989). The T cell repertoire and autoimmune diseases. *Annual Review of Immunology*, **7**, 657–82.

Lachmann, P. J. and Peters, D. K. (eds) (1982). *Clinical aspects of immunology*, (4th edn). Blackwell Scientific Publications, Oxford.

Lessof, M. H. (ed.) (1984). *Allergy. Immunological and clinical aspects*. Wiley, Chichester.

Miller, G. (ed.) (1986). *Autoimmunity. Immunological reviews*. Academic Press, Orlando.

Primary Immunodeficiency Diseases. Reports of a WHO Sponsored Meeting (1989). *Immunodeficiency Reviews*, **1**, 173–205.

Siegel, B. V. (1985). Immunology and oncology. *International Review of Cytology*, **96**, 89–120.

3

Monitoring the immune system

Experimentally, it is possible to critically measure the effects on immune function of many agents, and indeed the immunopharmacology of immunomodulating drugs has been largely defined in experimental animals. The situation is somewhat different in considering the effects in man. Clearly, there are toxicological considerations which have to be evaluated, and only drugs without significant toxic effects are suitable for clinical evaluation. However, if the drug is expected to modify the functions of the immune system as part of its therapeutic effect, then the ways in which this effect can be measured in man are limited.

The main methods of clinically evaluating the immune system are to assess the functions of peripheral blood cells, or to measure immunologically derived analytes in the blood plasma. Dclaycd type skin tests do give some indication of cellular immune function, but the number of antigens which are suited to this test is limited, and the results depend on a number of different, if interacting factors. Moreover, the antigens, once administered in a skin test, can theoretically modify the immune system in a specific manner, independent of any therapeutic agent, and hence changes in the tests when repeated may be difficult to evaluate.

The tests of immunological analytes in the blood include those which quantitatively measure antibodies, either as immunoglobulins or by their primary function of antigen combination.

Serum immunoglobulin levels

The three main immunoglobulins, IgG, IgA, and IgM are relatively easily measured in stored serum samples by well established immunochemical methods, many now automated. There are good standards and reagents available generally, and coefficients of variation of 5–10 per cent are readily achievable. The levels vary considerably with age, and the range in a healthy adult population is approximately 2.5 fold for IgG, and 4–5 fold for IgA and IgM.

Drugs which cause increased activity of the immune system seldom cause significant changes in the total levels of these proteins, neither does successful vaccination, since the proportion of the total immunoglobulin level attributable to any specific antibody activity is usually less than 1 per cent. On the other hand, increased catabolism may cause a fall in the serum levels, especially of IgG, and drugs which depress plasma cell differentiation may impair immunoglobulin synthesis generally, with resulting low levels of all the immunoglobulin classes. Some drugs have a more marked effect on some immunoglobulin classes than others, and selective depression of IgA has been reported with the anticonvulsant drug Phenytoin, and penicillamine used in the treatment of rheumatoid arthritis. However, these are unwanted side effects, and not part of the aims of therapy.

So-called immunosuppressive therapy for autoimmune disease, putatively aiming to depress the synthesis of harmful autoantibodies, often depresses immunoglobulin levels generally, so that both specific antibody activity and immunoglobulin levels may indicate effective therapy. However, the changes in immunoglobulin levels are not sufficiently constant to be reliable monitors of therapy.

Specific antibody activity

The measurement of specific antibodies is usually more relevant in the management of immunological diseases. In procedures to enhance antibody formation, such as vaccination, or to modify it, as in allergen immunotherapy, specific antibody is a necessary element in patient evaluation. In mass vaccination programmes this is of course impractical, but in the evaluation of vaccines, in clinical trials, some assessment of antibody responses is necessary, even if only in a representative sample of vaccinated individuals. Likewise, in trials of allergen immunotherapy, the changes in specific antibody of IgE and IgG classes are necessary to evaluate the clinical outcome. An increase in so-called 'blocking' antibodies of the IgG class is a common, but not invariable accompaniment of a successful clinical outcome of this procedure.

In diseases resulting from abnormal antibodies, usually autoantibodies, the effect of immunosuppressive therapy, including plasma exchange and treatment with steroids and cytotoxic drugs and agents, can often be seen by a reduction in the circulating antibody level. However, there may not be an absolute correlation between clinical benefit and reduction in serum antibody level, and this can be for a number of reasons:

(1) there may be other immunopathogenic factors such as those of cell-mediated immunity which operate independent of the antibody;

(2) for directly pathogenic antibodies it may be the tissue level of antibody which is important—the serum level is only the surplus, and changes in that may not closely follow changes in tissue levels;

(3) the antibody measured in the serum may be mainly epi-phenomenal, i.e. directed against antigens with minimal pathogenic effect.

Associated parameters of immunity

Changes in the complement system and the acute phase proteins occur during many immunological reactions. These can all be measured im-munochemically with some precision. The acute phase proteins (C-reactive protein, alpha-1 acid glycoprotein, haptoglobulin, etc.) do not measure any specific immunological process, but are usually elevated in inflammatory, traumatic, and neoplastic processes, and their return to normal values usually reflects clinical improvement. As such, they are non-specific parameters of effective therapy. Similarly, measure-ment of plasma levels of lymphokines (IL2, IL4, IL6) or of lymphokine receptors (IL2R) are coming into use as monitors of on-going immuno-logical activity.

The complement system is involved in many immunologically-mediated diseases including infection, of course, since it is activated by antigen–antibody complexes. However, since components of the sys-tem are usually acute phase proteins, changes in the plasma levels may be difficult to interpret as an effect of therapy. It is possible to measure the circulating breakdown products of activation of various com-ponents, especially C1, C3, C4 and the terminal C5–9 complex, and the levels of these 'activated' components (C3a, C3dg, C5a, etc.) in the circulation are often better measures of the involvement of the com-plement system in disease, and hence would be more suitable in the assessment of immunomodulating drugs. However, since the activation can occur readily *in vitro*, producing artefacts, logistic problems in specimen handling have to be overcome in any study.

Measurement of cell-mediated immunity

The main practical way of evaluating changes in cell-mediated immun-ity is by analysis of the peripheral blood lymphocytes. This can be done by analysis of cell surface markers for the expression of the antigens (CD2, CD3, CD4, etc.) indicative of functionally active cells, or by assessment of *in vitro* responsiveness of the cells when stimulated by non-specific activating substances (mitogens) such as phyto-haemagglutinin, or by specific antigens. This responsiveness can be assessed by measuring the degree of lymphokine (IL2 or gamma-interferon) produced, or the level of DNA synthesis as indicated by the incorporation of tritiated thymidine, or the amount of immunoglobu-lins or antibodies secreted into the tissue culture medium by the stimulated cells. Drugs and agents which enhance the immune response will lead to a normalization of the cell surface markers, as well as an increase in the functional parameters referred to above. On the other hand, immunosuppressive therapy may lead to a decline in the absolute and relative numbers of CD3 or CD4 positive cells, as well as decreased functional activity as assessed by *in vitro* methods.

However, these tests of cell-mediated immunity are time consuming and expensive in reagents and manpower, and present considerable logistic problems in the collection and transport of fresh blood samples to the centre where the specialized tests are performed. Also, while modern flow cytometry has automated cell surface marker analysis so that it is reasonably rapid and gives consistently reliable results, the functional tests are not nearly so robust, with considerable inter-assay variability. These factors, together with the inherent variability of some of these parameters in healthy individuals, has meant that relatively few trials of immunomodulating agents and procedures have been accompanied by data on changing parameters of cell-mediated immun-ity.

Suggested reading

Gooi, H. C. and Chapel, H. (1990). *Clinical immunology: a practical approach*. Oxford University Press, Oxford.

Hudson, L. and Hay, F. C. (1989). *Practical immunology*, (3rd edn). Black-well Scientific Publications, Oxford.

Rose, N. R., Friedman, H., and Fahey, J. L. (eds) (1986). *Manual of clinical laboratory immunology*. American Society for Microbiology, Washington D.C.

Thompson, R. A. (1981). *Techniques in clinical immunology*, (2nd edn). Blackwell Scientific Publications, Oxford.

Thompson, R. A. (1985). *Laboratory investigations of immunological dis-orders*. Clinics in Immunology and Allergy, Vol. 5, Number 3. W. B. Saun-ders, London.

4

Clinical trial methodology

Introduction

Clinical trials involving evaluation of the safety and efficacy of drugs which may ultimately be administered to millions of people represent one of the most important applications of the scientific method. However, the design of a valid clinical trial is quite subtle, and misleading results can easily be obtained with poor technique. In addition, clinical trial methodology is evolving. For example, new statistical procedures are available, such as sequential methods which permit the addition of each outcome to an ongoing analysis in order to recognize benefit or harm as early as possible. These methods, which have ethical as well as practical value, have been devised in such a way as to avoid the problems associated with repeated significance testing. Trial design is also evolving in order to cope with the testing of potential anti-HIV drugs. Such trials present a special set of problems of compliance and follow-up which must be solved if potential treatments or prophylactic measures are to be adequately investigated. Finally, it should not be forgotten that a clinical trial result, obtained in an adequately designed trial, provides rigorous confirmation of the original laboratory observations which gave rise to the drug being developed.

The principles and practice of clinical trial design and conduct have been set out very fully (Pocock 1983), and no attempt will be made here to emulate that excellent text in which can be found details of protocol design, trial rationale and ethics, informed consent, case report forms, data handling, and statistics.

The requirements of the American Food and Drug Administration (FDA), formalized as 'Good Clinical Research Practice (GCRP)' endeavour to apply rigorous quality control (QC) to clinical trials and to the subsequent handling of the data. These principles must be applied, unless any specific waivers are obtained from the FDA, in order for a trial to be accepted as pivotal data in a registration application for permission to market the drug in the USA. The central concept of GCRP is the 'data trail'. This is the route taken by information (e.g. symptom scores) from the patient via the medical notes and/or case report forms to the registration application documents. Quality control measures are aimed at reducing the probability of errors escaping unnoticed whenever the data is transcribed from one form to another. Data monitors regularly visit the trial hospital, audit the case report forms for completeness, discuss any illegible or puzzling data with the trialist, and, if permitted, compare the data on the case report forms with the data in the original patient notes. The activities of the data monitors are governed by 'Standard Operating Procedures (SOPs)' which set out his/her responsibilities. SOPs also govern all other aspects of trial design and conduct such as protocol preparation or the handling of adverse event reports. In this way, an outside agency can inspect the procedures used by a company and determine whether or not they are adequate to ensure that, for example, information about adverse events reaches the FDA. GCRP also has strict requirements about disclosure of financial remuneration and the means for obtaining informed consent. A set of guidelines for GCRP has been published by the Association of the British Pharmaceutical Industry (ABPI 1988).

The purpose of the present exercise has been to derive a list of features of trial design and conduct which were felt to be essential to a valid clinical trial, and to determine how far these criteria have been satisfied by a substantial number of the clinical trials of immunological agents conducted during the 1980s. In this way lessons can be learned and recommendations made for future trials. For clarity and uniformity, the chosen criteria were formalized into a scoring system.

The scoring system

Overview

Two versions of the scoring system were prepared, one for randomized control trials (RCTs) and one for studies without randomized controls (NRCTs). The latter system was therefore applied to a variety of study designs including:

(1) studies with historical controls;

(2) studies with no control group;

(3) studies in which the entire patient population received alternate periods of different treatments;

(4) studies in which the entire patient population received alternate periods of treatment and no treatment;

(5) studies in which patients were assigned to two or more parallel
treatment groups by a non-randomized procedure.

Copies of both scoring systems are included as appendices to this
chapter.

In the scoring system for RCTs, 32 questions were asked about each
trial covering study design (11 questions), the patient population (5
questions), drug administration (5 questions), patient monitoring (5
questions) and reporting and analysis (6 questions). The 'study design'
section included questions about randomization and blinding as well as
endpoints, stopping rules, and statistical aspects.

The scoring system was really no more than a checklist of the kind of
questions that should be asked when reading clinical trial papers with a
critical eye. Clearly, however, it would be impossible to read and
assimilate a couple of hundred papers and to be equally critical of each
without using a checklist. The scoring system is not based upon any
absolute indicators of quality, and it should be regarded principally as a
means of highlighting deficiencies rather than providing an accurate
credibility rating for each trial. Some readers will no doubt consider
that different aspects should be scored or given special emphasis, but
such changes will not alter the fact that the overall score achieved by a
trial represents only a very crude estimate of quality. It is intended that
the present scoring system, with all its imperfections, should serve to
stimulate constructive discussion of clinical trial methodology, rather
than debates about the precise scores achieved by particular studies
using this or any other scoring system.

The aim was to devise a scoring system which was not only
comprehensive but also 'user-friendly' in terms of simplicity. The
intention was to make each question as straightforward and unam-
biguous as possible in order to facilitate rapid but accurate assessment
of trial publications. Many of the questions simply asked whether an
item was reported or not, rather than requiring an opinion or judgement.
The range of responses to each question was limited to 'yes' (score 2),
'partial or ambiguous' (score 1), 'no' (score 0) and 'NA' (not applicable).
Some of the questions make unavoidable assumptions about the quality
of reporting of clinical trials. It has to be assumed, for example, that
when a primary endpoint is quoted in the 'methods' section of a paper,
this does not represent a *post-hoc* selection from a range of outcomes.
When scorable items were not described but reference was made to a
prior publication where the information can be found, the assigned
score refers to the item as presented in the referred publication.

Three categories of clinical trial were defined according to the score achieved—67 per cent or over ('high score'), 34–66 per cent ('grey area') and less than 34 per cent ('low score'). The 'grey area' concept was introduced because it seemed inappropriate to regard a study which achieved 49 per cent as 'low score' and one which achieved 51 per cent as 'high score' when the scoring system itself is not an absolute quantitative measure of quality.

Each question in the scoring system and its purpose is set out below. In all cases a definitive statement was required in order to avoid the default score of zero. For example, a statement that 'no adverse events were observed amongst the patients' would score '2', whereas an absence of any statement about adverse events, which could represent either a true absence or lax reporting, scored '0'. Similarly, a statement that the trial results were to be analysed on an 'intention-to-treat' basis scored '2' whereas an absence of any information about eligibility for analysis in terms of, for example, interrupted drug administration scored '0'.

The scoring system for RCTs

(A) Study design

1. Was there a primary efficacy endpoint? A statement of the hypothesis that the trialists set out to test is clearly essential to understanding the trial. Virtually no reports of clinical trials state the null hypothesis, for example: 'the trial was designed to test the hypothesis that there is no difference between the survival of patients on drug A and the survival of patients on drug B'. However, the purpose of the study should be clearly discernible in terms of a specific endpoint.

Statistical arguments indicate that the number of endpoints should be minimized. A p value of 0.05 implies there is a 1 in 20 chance of the null hypothesis being correct and a 19 in 20 chance that the observed difference between two treatments is a real difference. As the number of endpoints in a study increases, the greater the chance of a false difference having a p value of 0.05 and hence being erroneously regarded as a real difference. A score of 2 was therefore given for trials with a single endpoint and a score of 1 was given when there were two endpoints. Studies with more than two endpoints were given a score of zero. For the same reasons, stratified studies, in which the strata were separately evaluated, were scored as follows: one endpoint/two strata scored '1'; one endpoint/more than two strata scored '0'.

Various strategies are available for studies in which several endpoints are monitored. Some authors described one comparison as the major endpoint, around which the trial size had been determined, with the

remaining comparisons regarded as providing only exploratory or supportive data. Such studies scored '2'.

When the measurement of several variables is essential to determining whether or not a patient has responded, some form of combined
endpoint or index can be derived. An example of the former would be a
definition of a responding patient as one for whom each of four variables must exceed threshold values; if any of them fail to do so, then
the patient is a failure. An index takes the form of an equation that
derives one number from the values of the four variables, and this
number must exceed a threshold value for the patient to be considered
a responder.

Some studies involve the repeated measurement of a variable with
time. It is not correct to apply a statistical test at each time point
because of the danger of false positive results. There are various ways
of reducing the number of statistical tests. For example:

(1) comparing the time taken for each treatment group to attain a
    threshold value;

(2) comparing the time period over which each treatment group ex-
    ceeded a predetermined value;

(3) comparing data only at a predetermined time point;

(4) comparing the mean value, for the entire study period, for each
    treatment group.

2. Were the efficacy endpoint(s) defined?   It is essential that endpoints
are clearly defined in order to avoid confusion. For example, terms
such as 'partial remission of tumour' will be interpreted differently by
different trialists unless defined in terms of a percentage reduction in
tumour size as measured by a specified technique. Studies which made
quantitative observations and compared two groups of patients using,
for example, a *t*-test, did not involve the use of threshold levels. In such
cases the endpoint is defined by stating the method used to make the
measurements, unless universally standard methods were used (e.g.
haemoglobin level) which did not need further definition when 'NA'
was assigned. Methods were deemed worthy of stating if someone new
to the field (e.g. an immunologist) was unlikely to be familiar with
them. When the endpoint was death by any cause, this question
was assigned 'NA', but when the endpoint was death by a particular

cause then the criteria for establishing the cause of death must be stated.

3. Was informed consent obtained without knowledge of treatment allocation? The aim of randomization is to obtain comparable treatment groups. If patients know their treatment allocation before consent is requested, then the treatment groups can accrue quite different populations. For example, a patient who is severely ill might give consent for a treatment regimen which involves repeated lengthy infusions, whereas a patient with a milder form of the disease might consider that the ratio of potential benefit to inconvenience is too low. If the control group in the same trial involves a simpler regimen, such as two pills three times a day, then the latter type of patient may well give consent. The active treatment group thus acquires a more severely ill group of patients than the control group.

If the trialist is aware of treatment allocation then he is in a position to bias the enrolment into the treatment groups. An example of this would be a trialist giving a more encouraging account of the study when asking for informed consent from a more severely ill patient who has been randomized to the treatment which the clinician believes to be better. Thus one treatment group tends to acquire more serious cases, and may therefore show a reduced level of efficacy compared to the other group which accumulates less serious cases.

Double-blind trials always scored '2' for this question.

4. Was the randomization method described? Typically this involves the preparation by a third party of opaque, sealed envelopes bearing the patient number and containing a note of treatment allocation. Some form of random number generator is used by the third party to determine treatment allocation. One way of ensuring that informed consent is obtained before randomization is for the third party to supply the clinician with the envelope only in return for a signed informed consent document.

5. Were the patients blind to treatment allocation? See question 6.

6. Were the clinicians blind to treatment allocation? The degree of blinding is a valuable indicator of the weight that should be attached to a study, a higher degree of blinding giving a reduced opportunity for unintentional bias. Thus:

Type of trial	Score for question 5	Score for question 6	Total score
Double blind	2	2	4
'Improved' single blind*	2	1	3
Single blind	2	0	2
'Improved' open*	0	1	1
Open	0	0	0

* Patient managed by two doctors; one is aware of treatment allocation and administers the trial medication whilst the other is blind to treatment allocation and carries out the patient assessment.

7. Were both the patients and the clinicians blind to ongoing results for the trial as a whole?   It is harmful for the trialist to know of the ongoing result for the trial as a whole. Let us suppose that an interim analysis of a double blind trial shows a trend, that has not reached statistical significance, suggesting that one treatment is more effective than the other. The trialist may then find it difficult on ethical grounds to ask patients for consent to randomization if he believes that one treatment may be more beneficial. The trial may then grind to a halt, leaving a potentially valuable finding unsubstantiated. This illustrates the value of independent monitoring committees, equipped with pre-determined stopping rules, which are responsible for conducting interim analyses.

In open trials, awareness of ongoing results is more directly harmful, the trialist being in a position to bias the outcome by differential withdrawal of patients from the treatment groups. The final analysis of success and failure will therefore be insufficient without taking into account the withdrawn patients and the reasons for their withdrawal. If the randomization process is also not blinded, then the trialist who is aware of a trend favouring one treatment over the other is in a position to bias enrolment into the trial.

8. Were the statistical methods to be used in the analysis stated at the outset, and were they appropriate to the study design and the type of data being gathered?   Statistical methods are tools, each of which has been developed with a particular task in mind. Used inappropriately, unreliable results will be obtained. Statistical tests should be chosen at the initial planning stage of the trial in consultation with a professional statistician and with regard to both the type of data and the study design.

Life-table analysis and a logrank test, or a similar method (see below), should be used to analyse data involving the timecourse of events (e.g. deaths or tumour recurrences) rather than a simple comparison of the proportion of trial failures at one time point. Consider the statement: 'At 5 years there had been eight deaths amongst sixteen (50 per cent) patients enrolled on treatment A and ten deaths amongst twenty (50 per cent) patients enrolled on treatment B, not significant by Chi-square test'. This statement could conceal the fact that six patients on treatment A and three on treatment B were lost to follow-up or have yet to attain 5 years of trial participation. Such missing data is referred to as 'censorship'. Amongst the patients who attained 5 years of trial participation, the proportions would therefore be eight out of ten (80 per cent) mortality on drug A and ten out of seventeen (59 per cent) mortality on drug B. However, this does not make use of the data available on the nine patients who failed to reach 5 years of trial participation. It is also possible that the deaths on drug A mostly took place in the first 2 years, whereas the deaths on drug B took place mostly in the last 2 years. The use of life-table analysis, such as a Kaplan–Meier plot and a logrank test, is essential for this sort of data because it can cope with censorship and clearly portrays any differences in the timecourse of events. For summary purposes, the proportion of failures at a particular time point can be quoted but these will be the proportions derived from life-table analysis and will take account of censorship. Various other methods are available for the comparison of life-table data (e.g. Gehan 1965; Breslow 1970) although it is beyond the scope of this book to consider the relative merits of these methods. The Cox proportional hazards model is also available for analysing life-table data. This multivariate regression method takes into account baseline prognostic indicators. Christensen (1987) has reviewed this technique in fairly 'user friendly' terms.

Three basic choices which must be made when selecting a statistical method are between the use of 'paired' or 'unpaired' tests, 'one-sided' or 'two-sided' tests and 'parametric' or 'non-parametric' tests. Paired tests are used to compare data obtained on separate occasions from the same group of patients (e.g. baseline and post-treatment), whilst unpaired tests are used to compare data from independent sources. Two-sided tests, unlike one-sided tests, take into account both possible trial outcomes: that active treatment performs better than control *or* that active treatment performs worse than control. Two-sided tests are therefore routinely used in clinical trials. Non-parametric tests make far fewer assumptions about the distribution of the data than parametric tests and are therefore very useful when the distribution of the data is unknown. The well known parametric '*t*-test' is an adaption to small samples of a method for analysing normally distributed data. Essentially, the bell-shaped distribution curve flattens and broadens as the sample number reduces. It is not therefore appropriate if the distribution of the data is unknown or patently non-normal.

Study design features which influence the choice of statistics include the enrolment of patients into more than two treatment groups. For quantitative data, analysis of variance (ANOVA) will be required in order to avoid the dangers of false positives inherent in multiple comparisons. The Kruskal–Wallis method (Campbell 1989) is available for non-parametric data. For handling proportions, the Chi-square test can be performed on data from several treatment groups. For example, a 3 × 2 Chi-square test will compare two outcomes in three treatment groups. The data may then be further probed, according to rules decided upon before the start of the trial, for example: 'a 2 × 2 comparison of groups A and B will be performed if the 3 × 2 comparison of groups A, B and C indicates overall significance'. Specifying a very small number (one or two) of additional tests at the design stage of the trial helps to avoid accusations of 'data dredging'.

Some trials require each new result to be added to an ongoing analysis in order to watch for the conditions set out in a predetermined stopping rule. Sequential techniques, designed specifically for this purpose, must be used for such a trial (Whitehead 1983). It is not appropriate to simply carry out repeated significance tests on a large number of occasions. Sequential methods are being used increasingly often in studies on high-risk patients, in order to detect benefit or harm as quickly as possible. Such analyses are best carried out by monitoring committees who are unconnected with the trial sponsors or the hospital. The committee should include a professional statistician with experience in sequential methods. As an alternative to sequential methods, the committee could perform a small number of interim analyses seeking a much stricter level of significance on each occasion according to published methods (Pocock 1983).

Clearly, the best guide to statistics for the clinical trialist is to keep the design very simple and thus avoid the need for sophisticated statistical methodology. A statistician must be involved in the trial from the outset.

In order to score 2, the chosen statistical method must be stated in the 'Methods' section, accompanied by a sentence indicating how the method copes with the type of data and the study design. A 'NA' option was provided for the small number of studies which did not use any statistical methods.

9. Was the study multicentred? If so, was there provision for a check on the homogeneity of the data to ensure that one aberrant centre wasn't unduly influencing the results? This may take the form of a formal statistical analysis in the case of complex numerical data or a simple look at the proportion of successes, and sample number, for each centre.

10. Was the trial size determined at the outset by means of a statistical power calculation? It is essential that the size of a RCT is decided upon by means of a statistical power calculation so that the chance of a type two error (false negative) is known. The use of a predetermined trial size also avoids bias. If a horserace could be stopped at any stage, then the punters could more or less choose the winner. The decision as to which horse and jockey are the winning combination is made by having a predetermined endpoint. The same principle applies to clinical trials.

11. If the answer to question 10 was '0' (=no), was some other reason specified at the outset for the trial size? If the answer to question 10 was '2' or '1' and interim analyses were allowed, were stopping rules specified at the outset? Alternative reasons for the trial size include the number of patients becoming infected during an epidemic or, for some vaccine trials, the total population of a geographical region. When performing interim analyses, a statement at the outset of precise stopping rules avoids the form of bias described in question 10. An example would be a threshold ratio between the deaths in the test group and those in the control group.

(B) Patient population

12. Were the patient selection criteria clearly defined such that the trial could be repeated by other workers? Statements that, for example, 'patients with disease "x" were enrolled' are unsatisfactory. If the study did indeed take allcomers with a particular indication, regardless of severity and with no exclusions, then it is necessary to say so in order to score 2. Otherwise a list of qualifiers and exclusions (pregnancy, children, the elderly, concomitant diseases etc) is required.

13. Were the numbers of patients enrolled and evaluated in each treatment group/stratum etc. clearly stated? In order to facilitate a clear understanding of a set of results, it should not be necessary to perform mental arithmetic or make assumptions to establish these numbers from the paper. In an intention-to-treat study there will be no difference between the number enrolled and the number evaluated.

14. Was a record kept of the patients who were rejected and why? This refers to patients rejected because they did not fit the inclusion and/or exclusion criteria, prior to randomization. Such a record is essential in order to understand how far the trial population is representative of the general population with the disease of interest, and hence the potential breadth of application of the test drug. In the absence of a reject log the default score is 0, unless there is a statement that none were rejected, in which case the score is 2.

15. Was a list given of the patients who were withdrawn with reasons? This refers to patients who were randomized but whom the trialists subsequently excluded from the analysis. Such a log should be kept in order to show that any withdrawals were not made in a biased fashion. Whilst question 13 related to a record of the number of patients enrolled and evaluated (and hence withdrawn), this question refers to a listing of the reasons for withdrawal.

16. To what extent did the selected patients' general condition permit the detection of adverse events? (e.g. statements about the exclusion of patients with concomitant systemic disease) If patients are healthy in every way apart from the disease which is the subject of the trial, then it will be easier to spot adverse events. If, however, the patients have concomitant liver dysfunction of an exacerbating/remitting nature, for example, then it will be difficult to comment upon any adverse effects of the test drug upon liver function.

For a small number of trials, the disease which was the subject of the trial was of such a severe, disseminated form (e.g. septicaemia) that detection of adverse events would have been hampered. In such cases the assigned score was '0'.

Some of the AIDS trials which enrolled patients known to be indulging in substance abuse (e.g. drug addicts, glue-sniffers, etc.) scored '0' for this question.

(C) Drug administration

17. Was there an adequate description of the dosage regimen such that the trial could be repeated by other workers? A description of the dosage regimen in terms of quantity, route, frequency, duration, and special conditions such as restricted diet or activity is clearly essential. The sizes and timing of planned dosage changes (e.g. hyposensitization regimens) should be reported.

18. If the trial was conducted blind then was reference made to identity of the test drug and the comparator? If the patient or trialist is able to determine which treatment is which then the various forms of bias that attach to open studies become relevant. Sometimes considerations of identity must extend beyond simply the appearance or taste of the treatments. For example, a placebo-controlled study of interferon could be confounded by the routine induction of pyrexia by interferon but not by the placebo.

19. Was a record kept of any interruptions in drug administration and/or was there a stated policy for the inclusion or exclusion of such cases in the analysis? In any lengthy regimen, some patients will occasionally miss treatments. In order to avoid bias in the inclusion or exclusion of patients from the analysis, it is necessary to state at the outset a definition of an evaluable patient in terms of receipt of treatment. This may be very specific, such as: 'an evaluable patient is one who misses no more than 2 of the course of 52 injections'. Alternatively, the criterion may be pragmatic, recognizing that, in the real world, when the drug is in routine medical use, injections will be missed: 'The intention is to test the efficacy of this regimen regardless of any gaps in administration that may occur' (i.e. 'intention-to-treat' trials). A 'NA' option was provided for trials involving only a single administration.

20. Was a specific statement made concerning the exclusion of other treatments likely to influence immune status or the attainment of trial endpoints, prior to and during the trial period? A knowledge of the other therapies received by trial patients is essential to interpreting the results of the study.

21. Did the study include a treatment crossover? If so, was the possibility of a 'carry-over effect' considered? Data should be provided or referred to that supports the length of the washout period in terms of drug persistence and longevity of the treatment effect. It is not sufficient to rely upon, for example, the half-life of a drug in blood because the biological effects of a drug may persist long after it has become undetectable. This is probably the case for many immunotherapeutic agents, because they activate cellular processes which may take weeks or months to be completed. Provision may be made for analysing the data for carry-over effects (Pocock 1983).

(D) Patient monitoring

22. How objective were the clinical monitoring methods? In general, the following scheme was applied, any variations being discussed at the appropriate point in the text.

physical measurement (e.g. lung function or the size of a readily accessible and discrete lesion) scored 2;

clinical assessment in terms of ordinal data (e.g. mild/moderate/severe categorization) is subject to inter-observer variation and scored 1;

clinical assessment in terms of ordinal data performed by two or more independent observers and the reporting of mean data scored 2;

reliance solely upon a patient's subjective perception of his symptoms, reported verbally, scored 0;

reliance solely upon a patient's subjective perception of his symptoms, as recorded on a daily basis using a simple predetermined scale, commencing with a period of baseline measurements prior to trial therapy and organized such that the patient cannot see his previous input scored 1.

23. Were measures of immunological function used which were relevant to the immunological aspect of the disease? This question concerns only tests of immune *function*. Simple enumeration of cells (e.g. CD3, CD4 etc) was not considered and studies using only these methods were assigned 'NA'.

Many trials report only tests of non-specific mitogen responsiveness or skin reactions to some common antigens. Whilst this is appropriate in some cases, in many others there are particular features of the immune system which have a special relevance to the disease of interest and which are suitable for routine monitoring (e.g. specific antibody responses or non-specific NK cell activity). The nature of the relevant tests varied between the therapeutic areas surveyed, and so the scoring criteria for this question are set out in each of the following chapters. As a general rule, however, '0' was scored when immune function was assessed using general methods of no direct relevance to the disease of interest. '2' was assigned when a range of relevant tests was employed.

24. Is there reference to close monitoring for adverse events in terms of questioning of patients and laboratory tests? The concept of the 'adverse event' replaced the term 'side-effect' some years ago because the causal relationship between drug and event may not be immediately apparent. The classic example is a patient falling and breaking his leg. This could be either a random event or an effect of the drug upon the patient's balance or bone strength. In principle, long term monitoring of many patients for adverse events, whether patently drug-related or not, will ultimately reveal correlations which might suggest causality.

However, the practicalities and considerable limitations of such surveillance, extending into the post-marketing phase, are beyond the scope of this book.

For the present scoring system, it was assumed that there had been questioning of patients if subjective symptoms such as pain, nausea, or fatigue were reported. Laboratory tests included hepatic function tests, renal function tests, and differential blood counts.

25. Was the possibility of adverse immunological events commented upon? As Chapter 1 makes clear, the immune system is a complex network of cells and soluble mediators which is not yet fully understood. There are not only mechanisms responsible for eliminating infection but also mechanisms by which tolerance is maintained towards self antigens or can be induced towards certain foreign antigens. Many immunotherapeutic agents interact with this system at several points in the network, and produce a constellation of effects which are also not yet fully characterized. Not all of these effects may be desirable. It is therefore appropriate, in clinical trials, to look for any potentially harmful immunological events, such as the rejection of previously stable transplants or the appearance of autoimmune phenomena in patients being treated with immunostimulants. Alternatively, immunosuppressants could increase the incidence or severity of concomitant infections or even provide a 'window of opportunity' for neoplasms to escape surveillance and become established. Hyposensitization therapy is associated with the risk of life-threatening systemic anaphylaxis. The transient reduction in some cell counts induced by interferon and the local skin reactions following administration of agents such as BCG were included in this question.

26. If the study was multicentred, were steps taken to standardize clinical and laboratory evaluations? Examples would include: periodic meetings of all investigators to review each patient's results and to reach a consensus on success or failure; review of all patients' outcomes by an independent committee; processing of blood samples from all participating hospitals at a single laboratory. If the endpoints were indisputable (e.g. death by any cause) or involved routine methods with existing QC (e.g. haemoglobin level) then the question was scored as 'NA'.

(E) Reporting and analysis

27. Were the pretreatment values for clinical and immunological variables fully presented and analysed? This is necessary in order to demonstrate comparability of treatment groups (success of randomization)

and to provide a firm database for assessing treatment effects. Reports
of prophylactic trials must include evidence that the treatment groups
were equally exposed to the disease-provoking agent.

28. Were the results fully and clearly presented?   In order to facilitate
an understanding of the results, there should be no need for assumptions or complicated mental arithmetic. The time points at which the
results were obtained should be clearly stated.

   Subgroups or pooled results, derived *post-hoc*, should not be reported as the main result. Such data can only be suggestive of another
clinical trial and can never be regarded as a firm outcome. To understand this, let us suppose the judges at Wimbledon, as well as comparing the total scores achieved by the players in a match, were at liberty
to compare, using statistical tests, the performance of the players
according to a range of secondary criteria such as the relative number
of points scored when the sun was shining, when it was cloudy, and
when cheering could be heard from the adjacent court. They might well
find, whilst the differential between the players was minimal in the
match as a whole, it was marked when the sun was shining. There are a
number of problems inherent in concluding that one player is better
than the other in the sunshine. Firstly, assuming the number of shots
played in the sunshine was less than the number of shots played in the
match as a whole, the apparently better performance of one player may
simply reflect a chance result in a small sample. Secondly, the chance of
spurious statistical significance increases with the number of endpoints
tested. Finally, the element of bias is represented by the judges knowing
that one player has better visual adaption to bright light than the other.
If this player were proclaimed the winner even though the overall result
(the planned endpoint) was a tie, the other player would be understand-
ably upset. In the same way, it is absurd to claim, for example, that a
drug is better than the control treatment because fewer patients with
duodenal ulcers died if in fact the planned endpoint had been the
mortality amongst patients with all forms of gastro-intestinal bleeding.

*29. Was the incidence of adverse events in each treatment group and their
severity and duration clearly stated?*   This is clearly essential for determining the relative safety of two treatments. It is most important that
severity and duration are reported as well as the outcome of any
measures taken to alleviate adverse symptoms.

30. Were the drop-outs and censored patients dealt with appropriately?
There are many reasons why patients may fail to complete their partici-

pation in a trial. They may be withdrawn by the trialists (question 15) because of protocol violation, adverse events or lack of efficacy. Some withdraw themselves and the reason may never be determined. Some may default because the treatment is not working, in which case differential loss to follow-up from the treatment groups may bias the result if the drop-outs are not included in the overall analysis. Others may drop out because of subjective side-effects or difficulties with drug administration (e.g. too complicated a procedure). Efforts should be made to re-contact drop-outs in order to obtain a reason for their discontinuing trial participation.

It is essential that the number of drop-outs in each treatment group is clearly reported as well as the stage of the trial at which they were censored. For Kaplan–Meier plots this can be achieved by indicating at several time-points on the graph the number of patients per group who are still at risk of trial failure.

The last known result for the censored patients should be included in the efficacy analysis unless a protocol criterion, specified at the outset of the trial, has been violated, for example: 'patients will be included in the analysis if they complete at least 3 months of treatment'. Such a criterion would be justified if, for example, there were strong grounds for believing that the drug being tested only exerts its effects after 3 months. In such a case, the reasons for censorship prior to 3 months should still be reported. If it were found, for example, that a large number of patients withdrew before 3 months because of an unacceptable side-effect then the value of the drug is diminished, no matter how convincing the efficacy observed after 3 months in the remaining patients.

The number of censored patients in each treatment group and the reasons for censorship should be compared, and any pattern commented upon.

The complete exclusion of drop-outs from the main analysis, without a separate analysis of the withdrawn group, is not acceptable, and scored '0'.

31. Were the statistical analyses fully reported? Particularly important features of statistical reporting are:

(i) For 'mean $+/-x$' it should be stated whether 'x' was the standard deviation or the standard error of the mean;

(ii) The name of the statistical test used should be quoted adjacent to p values unless it is categorically stated in the 'Methods' section that only one statistical method was used throughout the trial.

(iii) An exact *p* value should be given, not just a statement such as 'not significant' or '*p* <0.05'. The importance of this is illustrated by the statement: 'In a trial with three treatment groups, the incidence of side-effect "X" in treatment group "A" was "not significant" compared to the control group, whilst comparison of treatment group "B" with the control group yielded *p* <0.05'. Clearly this could be a dangerous statement if the *p* value for the first comparison was 0.055 and for the second it was 0.045. *P* = 0.05 is wrongly regarded as some kind of magical threshold whereby results have quite different properties on either side of this value. On the contrary, the *p* value represents the probability of the observed difference being due to chance. It follows that both of the comparisons above, if they did indeed have the values suggested, would be worrying.

(iv) Confidence intervals should be quoted as well as *p* values, and have been required in order to qualify for publication in the *British Medical Journal* since 1 July 1986. The importance of confidence intervals has been discussed by several authors (Langman 1986; Gardner and Altman 1986; Evans *et al.* 1988). Essentially, confidence intervals provide a way of escaping from the narrow thinking, discussed in (iii) above, that a result is meaningful only if it passes the threshold of a statistical significance test such as *p* = 0.05. Confidence intervals also carry much more information than is conveyed by quoting the mean results for two treatment groups and a *p* value. Confidence intervals give an indication of the range of values that could be expected for the mean in repeat studies. Suppose the observed difference in the value of a clinical variable between two treatment groups was found to be − 10. Let us further suppose this difference has a *p* value of 0.04 and a clinically meaningful difference was considered to be a decrease of 7. To what extent should the result of this trial be regarded as clinically significant? The answer is given by calculating the confidence interval for the difference between the means. If the confidence interval was found to extend from − 7 to − 13 then the result would appear to be important. If, however, the confidence interval extended from − 2 to −18, then the possibility would exist that a repeat trial would yield a result with no clinical significance.

32. Was the result discussed in terms of the trial size?   A clinical trial is a statistical sampling exercise in which the reliability of the result depends upon the size of the sample. The result should therefore be discussed in terms of the trial size.

For trials in which no power calculation was performed at the outset and no difference was observed between the active and control treatments, a *post-hoc* power calculation should be performed and the possibility of type II error discussed.

When a power calculation was performed at the outset but no difference was observed between the treatments, possible reasons for the differences between observed and expected results should be discussed. Commonly the control group does better than expected. This may be due to the 'placebo effect' of the trial patients having more attention lavished upon them than would normally be the case for non-trial patients.

When a power calculation was performed at the outset and the projected results were indeed observed, this question was assigned 'NA'.

Finally, when no statistical reason was given for the trial size but a statistically significant difference was observed between the treatment groups, the trialists should comment upon the reliability of their results in terms of the sample size. Confidence intervals are very relevant here in terms of, for example, the results discussed in question 31 above. The confidence interval narrows as the size of the sample of patients increases. Thus the confidence interval is a mathematical statement of the often quoted expression: 'this result is interesting but must be confirmed in larger studies'.

The scoring system for NRCTs

The scoring system for NRCTs consisted of 28 questions covering study design (8 questions), the patient population (5 questions), drug administration (5 questions), patient monitoring (5 questions) and reporting and analysis (5 questions).

As before, three categories of clinical trial were defined according to the score achieved—67 per cent or over ('high score'), 50–66 per cent ('grey area') and less than 50 per cent ('low score'). Note that the threshold between 'grey area' and 'low score' was set higher than for RCTs.

The scoring system for NRCTs was essentially the same as that for RCTs with the following changes. Questions 3 and 4, relating to randomization, were deleted. The questions relating to blindness were given 'NA' options for non-comparative trials, as also was question 1, concerning the number of endpoints. Questions 10, 11 and 32 relating to trial size and power calculations were replaced by one question asking simply: 'Was a reason given for the size of the trial?' The reason for the number of patients enrolled into a NRCT is virtually never given in publications. It is, however, an important point because in some studies the overall proportion of responding patients would have been quite different had the trial stopped with, for example, two or three or four fewer patients. It is perhaps reasonable to accept that a study with ten or twenty patients probably represents a planned trial size, but why do so many NRCTs have seven or thirteen patients? How much weight should be attached to a study where the proportion of responding patients was four out of thirteen (31 per cent), when it is apparent from the chronological list of patient data that the proportion of responders would have been 10 per cent if recruitment had ceased at ten patients. The ever present danger of bias is represented here by the publication of a set of results when they look sufficiently impressive rather than when a predetermined number of cases have been investigated.

Quality control questions

A further series of questions were applied to 'grey-area' and 'high-score' trials relating to quality control of the data. These supplementary questions, which did not contribute to the main score, were as follows:

(i)   Was mention made of the auditing of case report forms or QC of data recording and handling procedures in general?

(ii) Were any tests carried out to check the blinding of clinicians or laboratory staff by, for example, asking them which treatment group they think a number of patients were in? Were the patients asked, at the end of their trial participation, which group they think they were in?

(iii) Were compliance tests reported (e.g. counting of returned pills) in studies involving self-administration of drugs by out-patients (or administration by a family member)?

(iv) If the study was multicentred and the laboratory tests were performed centrally, was the system for transporting samples to the monitoring laboratory tested for deterioration of the sample (e.g. the effect of 24–48 hours at room temperature in the postal system)?

Power calculations

As part of this survey, power calculations were performed for 'grey-area' or 'high-score' RCTs whenever these were not provided by the trialists and no statistical difference was observed between the treatment groups.

Power calculations were only performed on 'qualitative' data, in the form of the proportions which did or did not achieve an endpoint (e.g. percentage mortality). The calculation of power for such data requires only that the proportions of successes and failures be known. By contrast, the calculation for quantitative data requires an estimate of the standard deviation for both groups and the data should be, at least approximately, normally distributed. Most studies which produced quantitative data, however, included no indication of the data distribution, and many trialists used non-paramctric statistics which do not provide an estimate of the standard deviation. Individual patient data, allowing calculation of the standard deviation, was not usually provided within the space constraints of the publication.

Power was calculated assuming a repeat trial was to be performed using the same number of patients and anticipating the same level of success in the control group as in the published trial. Only very rarely did the trialists state the level of success in the treatment group which would be considered a *clinically* significant improvement, as opposed to a statistically significant improvement, over the control group. The calculations were therefore performed in such a way as to determine the level of success in the treatment group for which the power of the trial would be 80 per cent.

The method of Pocock (1983) was applied:

$$N = \frac{[p_1 (100-p_1) + p_2 (100-p_2)]}{(p_1 - p_2)^2} \times f(a,b)$$

where:

$f(a,b)$ = a function of the desired levels of significance and power. The desired level of statistical significance was assumed to be $p = 0.05$ throughout and the level of power sought was 80 per cent. The corresponding value of $f(a,b)$ was 7.9.

N = the number of patients per treatment group. When the published trial had treatment groups of unequal size, the number of patients in the smallest group was used in the calculations as 'N'.

p_2 = the published percentage of successes in the control group.

p_1 = the percentage of successes in the treatment group. This was calculated using the foregoing values for $f(a,b)$, N and p_2.

Limitations included:

1. The use of $p = 0.05$ as the desired level of significance ignores the need for a stricter level of significance in some studies where interim analyses are desirable or multiple comparisons cannot be avoided.

2. The calculations are limited to 2×2 comparisons. For trials with more than two groups of patients (e.g. treatment groups A and B and control group C) separate power calculations were performed for each treatment group versus the control group (i.e. A *versus* C and B *versus* C). For trials with one immunotherapy group and two or more control groups (e.g. a chemotherapy group and a 'no-treatment' group) power was calculated for the comparison of immunotherapy with the group which received the least trial medication (i.e. the 'no-treatment' group in the example cited).

3. Had the calculation been performed by the trialists before commencing the published trial, they might well have anticipated a rather different level of success in the control group from that actually observed and used in this calculation.

4. The calculation did not take account of the fact that some reported proportions were derived from life-table analyses rather than having been obtained at a single time-point. The published tables of Freedman (1982), which provide the number of patients required for trials employing such analyses, were used in such cases to supplement the above calculations. However, the outcome was not substantially different from that obtained with the method above, and the results of using the Freedman method are not reported here.

Despite the limitations and imperfections of these calculations, they give a reasonable guide to the proportion of trials which were of sufficient size to detect as significant a clinically useful level of benefit for the test drug.

Appendix 4.1: Scoring system for randomized control trials

	Score	Possible scores[*]
A: Study design		
1. Was there a primary efficacy endpoint?	—	2 or 1 or 0
2. Were the efficacy endpoint(s) defined?	—	2 or 1 or 0 or NA
3. Was informed consent obtained without knowledge of treatment allocation?	—	2 or 1 or 0
4. Was the randomization method described?	—	2 or 1 or 0

[*]2 = yes, good etc; 1 = partial, reported for some results but not others, ambiguous etc; 0 = no, poor, not done, etc. *or* insufficient information given to permit judgement; NA = not applicable.

	Score	Possible scores[*]
5. Were the patients blind to treatment allocation?	—	2 or 1 or 0
6. Were the clinicians blind to treatment allocation?	—	2 or 1 or 0
7. Were both the patients and the clinicians blind to ongoing results for the trial as a whole?	—	2 or 1 or 0
8. Were the statistical methods to be used in the analysis stated at the outset and were they appropriate to the study design and the type of data being gathered?	—	2 or 1 or 0 or NA
9. Was the study multicentred? If so, was there provision for a check on the homogeneity of the data to ensure that one aberrant centre wasn't unduly influencing the results?	—	2 or 1 or 0 or NA
10. Was the trial size determined at the outset by means of a statistical power calculation?	—	2 or 1 or 0
11. If the answer to question 10 was '0' (= no), was some other reason specified at the outset for trial size? If the answer to question 10 was '2' or '1' and interim analyses were allowed, were stopping rules specified at the outset?	—	2 or 1 or 0 or NA

B: Patient population

12. Were the patient selection criteria clearly defined such that the trial could be repeated by other workers?	—	2 or 1 or 0
13. Were the numbers of patients enrolled and evaluated in each treatment group/ stratum etc clearly stated?	—	2 or 1 or 0
14. Was a record kept of the patients who were rejected and why?	—	2 or 1 or 0
15. Was a list given of the patients who were withdrawn with reasons?	—	2 or 1 or 0 or NA
16. To what extent did the selected patients' general condition permit the detection of adverse events? (e.g. statements about the exclusion of patients with concomitant systemic disease).	—	2 or 1 or 0

Appendix 4.1: *(contd.)*

	Score	Possible scores[*]
C: Drug administration		
17. Was there an adequate description of the dosage regimen such that the trial could be repeated by other workers?	—	2 or 1 or 0
18. If the trial was conducted blind then was reference made to identity of the test drug and the comparator?	—	2 or 1 or 0 or NA
19. Was a record kept of any interruptions in drug administration? Was there a stated policy for the inclusion or exclusion of such cases in the analysis?	—	2 or 1 or 0 or NA
20. Was a specific statement made concerning the exclusion of other treatments likely to influence immune status or the attainment of trial endpoints, prior to and during the trial period?	—	2 or 1 or 0
21. Did the study include a treatment crossover? If so, was the possibility of a 'carry-over' effect considered?	—	2 or 1 or 0 or NA
D: Patient monitoring		
22. How objective were the clinical monitoring methods?	—	2 or 1 or 0
23. Were measures of immunological function used which were relevant to the immunological aspect of the disease?	—	2 or 1 or 0 or NA
24. Is there reference to close monitoring for adverse events in terms of questioning of patients and laboratory tests?	—	2 or 1 or 0
25. Was the possibility of adverse immunological events commented upon?	—	2 or 1 or 0
26. If the study was multicentred, were steps taken to standardize clinical and laboratory evaluations?	—	2 or 1 or 0 or NA

[*]2 = yes, good etc; 1 = partial, reported for some results but not others, ambiguous etc; 0 = no, poor, not done, etc. *or* insufficient information given to permit judgement; NA = not applicable.

	Score	Possible scores[*]
E: Reporting and analysis		
27. Were the pretreatment values for clinical and immunological parameters fully presented and analysed?	—	2 or 1 or 0
28. Were the results fully and clearly presented?	—	2 or 1 or 0
29. Was the incidence of adverse events in each treatment group and their duration and severity clearly stated?	—	2 or 1 or 0
30. Were the drop-outs and censored patients dealt with appropriately?	—	2 or 1 or 0 or NA
31. Were the statistical analyses fully reported?	—	2 or 1 or 0 or NA
32. Was the result discussed in terms of the trial size?	—	2 or 1 or 0 or NA
TOTAL SCORE:	—	
TOTAL POSSIBLE SCORE: = (32 minus the number of NA questions) × 2		$= (32 - \underline{\quad}) \times 2 = \underline{\quad}$
PERCENTAGE SCORE:	—	

Quality control (QC)
(not part of the main score)

(i) Was mention made of the auditing of case report forms or QC of data recording and handling procedures in general?	—	yes/no
(ii) Were any tests carried out to check the blinding of clinicians or laboratory staff by, for example, asking them which treatment group they think a number of patients were in? Were the patients asked, at the end of their trial participation, which group they think they were in?	—	yes/no/NA
(iii) Were compliance tests reported (e.g. counting of returned pills) in studies involving self-administration of drugs by out-patients (or administration by a family member)?	—	yes/no/NA

[*] 2 = yes, good etc; 1 = partial, reported for some results but not others, ambiguous etc; 0 = no, poor, not done, etc. *or* insufficient information given to permit judgement; NA = not applicable.

Appendix 4.1: *(contd.)*

	Score	Possible scores[*]
(iv) If the study was multicentred and the laboratory tests were performed centrally, was the system for transporting samples to the monitoring laboratory tested for deterioration of the sample (e.g. the effect of 24–48 hours at room temperature in the postal system)?	—	yes/no/NA
Summary statement: Were the applicable QC checks performed?	—	YES/SOME/NO

[*]NA = not applicable.

Trial summary:
Test drug:
Control drug:
Patient numbers:
Test drug benefit:
Disease:
Aim:
Statistical methods:
Clinical methods:
Immunological methods:
Any correlation between clinical and immunological results?

Appendix 4.2: Scoring system for trials without randomized controls

	Score	Possible scores[*]
A: Study design		
1. Was there a primary endpoint?	—	2 or 1 or 0 or NA
2. Were the efficacy endpoint(s) defined?	—	2 or 1 or 0 or NA
3. Was there a concurrent control group? If so, were the patients blind to treatment allocation?	—	2 or 1 or 0 or NA
4. Was there a concurrent control group? If so, were the clinicians blind to treatment allocation?	—	2 or 1 or 0 or NA

	Score	Possible scores[*]
5. Was there a concurrent control group? If so, were both the patients and the clinicians blind to ongoing results?	—	2 or 1 or 0 or NA
6. Were the statistical methods to be used in the analysis stated at the outset and were they appropriate to the study design and the type of data being gathered?	—	2 or 1 or 0 or NA
7. Was the study multicentred? If so, was there provision for a check on the homogeneity of the data to ensure that one aberrant centre wasn't unduly influencing the results?	—	2 or 1 or 0 or NA
8. Was a reason given for the size of the trial?	—	2 or 1 or 0

B: Patient population

9. Were the patient selection criteria clearly defined such that the trial could be repeated by other workers?	—	2 or 1 or 0
10. Were the numbers of patients enrolled and evaluated (in each group or stratum if appropriate) clearly stated?	—	2 or 1 or 0
11. Was a record kept of the patients who were rejected and why?	—	2 or 1 or 0
12. Was a list given of the patients who were withdrawn with reasons?	—	2 or 1 or 0 or NA
13. To what extent did the selected patients' general condition permit the detection of adverse events? (e.g. statements about the exclusion of patients with concomitant systemic disease).	—	2 or 1 or 0

C: Drug administration:

14. Was there an adequate description of the dosage regimen such that the trial could be repeated by other workers?	—	2 or 1 or 0
15. If the trial was conducted blind then was reference made to identity of the test drug and the comparator?	—	2 or 1 or 0 or NA

[*]2 = yes, good etc; 1 = partial, reported for some results but not others, ambiguous etc; 0 = no, poor, not done, etc. *or* insufficient information given to permit judgement; NA = not applicable.

Appendix 4.2: *(contd.)*

	Score	Possible scores[*]
16. Was a record kept of any interruptions in drug administration? Was there a stated policy for the inclusion or exclusion of such cases in the analysis?	—	2 or 1 or 0 or NA
17. Was a specific statement made concerning the exclusion of other treatments likely to influence immune status or the attainment of trial endpoints, prior to and during the trial period?	—	2 or 1 or 0
18. Did the study include a treatment crossover? If so, was the possibility of a 'carry-over' effect considered?	—	2 or 1 or 0 or NA
D: Patient monitoring		
19. How objective were the clinical monitoring methods?	—	2 or 1 or 0
20. Were measures of immunological function used which were relevant to the immunological aspect of the disease?	—	2 or 1 or 0 or NA
21. Is there reference to close monitoring for adverse events in terms of questioning of patients and laboratory tests?	—	2 or 1 or 0
22. Was the possibility of adverse immunological events commented upon?	—	2 or 1 or 0
23. If the study was multicentred, were steps taken to standardize clinical and laboratory evaluations?	—	2 or 1 or 0 or NA
E: Reporting and analysis		
24. Were the pretreatment values for clinical and/or immunological parameters fully presented and analysed?	—	2 or 1 or 0
25. Were the results fully and clearly presented?	—	2 or 1 or 0
26. Was the incidence of adverse events (in each treatment group if appropriate) and their duration and severity clearly stated?	—	2 or 1 or 0

[*]2 = yes, good etc; 1 = partial, reported for some results but not others, ambiguous etc; 0 = no, poor, not done, etc. *or* insufficient information given to permit judgement; NA = not applicable.

	Score	Possible scores[*]
27. Were the drop-outs and censored patients dealt with appropriately?	—	2 or 1 or 0 or NA
28. Were the statistical analyses fully reported?	—	2 or 1 or 0 or NA
TOTAL SCORE:	—	
TOTAL POSSIBLE SCORE: (28 minus the number of NA questions) × 2		$= (28 - \underline{}) \times 2 = \underline{}$
PERCENTAGE SCORE:	—	

Quality control (QC)
(not part of the main score)

	Score	Possible scores
(i) Was mention made of the auditing of case report forms or QC of data recording and handling procedures in general?	—	yes/no
(ii) Were any tests carried out to check the blinding of clinicians or laboratory staff by, for example, asking them which treatment they think a number of patients were on? Were the patients asked, at the end of their trial participation, which treatment they think they were on?	—	yes/no/NA
(iii) Were compliance tests reported (e.g. counting of returned pills) in studies involving self-administration of drugs by out-patients (or administration by a family member)?	—	yes/no/NA
(iv) If the study was multicentred and the laboratory tests were performed centrally, was the system for transporting samples to the monitoring laboratory tested for deterioration of the sample (e.g. the effect of 24–48 hours at room temperature in the postal system)?	—	yes/no/NA
Summary statement: Were the applicable QC checks performed?	—	YES/SOME/NO

[*]2 = yes, good etc; 1 = partial, reported for some results but not others, ambiguous etc; 0 = no, poor, not done, etc. *or* insufficient information given to permit judgement; NA = not applicable.

Trial summary:
Test drug:
Control drug:
Patient numbers:
Test drug benefit:
Disease:
Aim:
Statistical methods:
Clinical methods:
Immunological methods:
Any correlation between clinical and immunological results?

5

Immunotherapeutic approaches to cancer

Introduction

The application of immunotherapy as a fourth modality for the treatment of cancer is based on the premise that the immune system is capable of recognizing and destroying tumour cells. Just as the immune system maintains constant surveillance for infection and acts both specifically and non-specifically to destroy pathogens, so it has been proposed that tumours arise with high frequency in the healthy individual and are eradicated by an ever vigilant immune response. Such a theory could explain why the probability of contracting cancer increases with age as the immune system becomes less efficient. Yet cancer can occur in the absence of any detectable immune deficiency, and this has led to the notion that the tumour somehow blocks the action of the immune effector mechanisms which attempt to destroy it. Recognition of a tumour could be either specific or non-specific, depending upon the changes which take place on the surface of a cell when it is transformed to the cancerous state. It is possible to envisage tumour-specific antigens which are unique to particular types of cancer or, alternatively, changes which are common to every kind of cancer cell regardless of origin. Beverley (1983) has provided a critical review of the methods used to probe for the existence of specific tumour-cell antigens and specific T-lymphocyte-mediated responses. The complexity of the immune system ensures that the classic biological problem of reconciling *in vitro* with *in vivo* events is paramount. Just because a particular type of cell is capable of a potentially useful trick in cell culture gives no indication of the quantitative relevance of this mechanism during the normal *in vivo* response. At least four possible immune mechanisms may be involved in tumour eradication, two of which are antigen specific and two are not. The specific mechanisms involve the recognition of tumour surface antigens by either B- or T-lymphocytes and the production of antibodies or the generation of a direct cytotoxic response, respectively. Anti-tumour antibodies could mediate tumour eradication either by Antibody Dependent Cellular Cytotoxicity (ADCC) or by the complement system. ADCC is effected by Natural Killer (NK) cells which attach to the Fc region of antibodies when they attach to cell surface antigen. Non-specific tumour cytotoxicity is mediated directly by NK cells as well as monocytes. These presumably attach to a molecule which is common to the cell surface of all tumours. Gangliosides have been suggested as the site for NK attachment.

Whatever the precise mechanism, the aims of immunotherapy are to induce tumour regression, to maintain remission, and to prolong survival. Immunotherapy is usually used as an adjunct to surgery, chemotherapy, or radiotherapy. Reasons for using immunotherapy alone include an inoperable location or type of tumour (e.g. some brain tumours; disseminated micro-metastases; leukaemia) and evidence that other methods do not work or have unacceptable side-effects. For example, the general condition of a patient may make them unsuitable candidates for the rigours of chemotherapy. A further use for immunotherapy is to counter the immunosuppressive effects of the other treatments and thus reduce the incidence of serious infection and/or permit more aggressive chemotherapy. Finally, immunotherapy may be used to accelerate the re-establishment of bone marrow transplants. Removal of a sample of bone marrow prior to chemotherapy and its replacement afterwards is being tested as a way of avoiding the myelo-suppression associated with aggressive chemotherapy. The period immediately following reimplantation is associated with a high level of neutropaenia and infection, and trials are underway with immunotherapeutic agents in an attempt to alleviate these events.

Outcome of scoring

Overview

Eighty clinical trials were assessed, of which thirty-three were RCTs involving 4267 evaluable patients and 47 were NRCTs involving 1634 evaluable patients.

RCTs

The RCT scores ranged from 24 per cent to 68 per cent, with a median of 35 per cent and a mean of 37 per cent. There was no evidence for the quality of the trials improving with time. The scores achieved by the RCTs were tested for correlation with year of publication and none was found ($R^2 = 0.130$). Table 5.1 shows the distribution of scores amongst

Table 5.1   Score frequencies for each question (RCTs)

Question number	Subject of question	Score frequency (per cent)			Sample* number
		2	1	0	
Questions which usually scored '2'					
8	Choice of statistical methods	42.42	18.18	39.39	33
12	Reporting of patient selection criteria	78.79	21.21	0.00	33
13	Reporting of patient numbers	66.67	30.30	3.03	33
17	Reporting of dosage regimen	66.67	33.33	0.00	33
22	Objectivity of clinical monitoring	63.64	30.30	6.06	33
23	Relevance of immunological monitoring	42.86	28.57	28.57	7
24	Close monitoring for adverse events	36.36	36.36	27.27	33
27	Baseline comparison of patients	51.52	27.27	21.21	33
28	Reporting of results	57.58	27.27	15.15	33
Questions which usually scored '1'					
15	Patient withdrawal log	36.36	45.45	18.18	22
29	Adverse event reporting	33.33	45.45	21.21	33
31	Statistical reporting	9.09	48.48	42.42	33
Questions which usually scored '0'					
1	Number of endpoints	15.15	27.27	57.58	33
2	Definition of endpoints	33.33	30.30	36.36	33
3	Informed consent before randomization	15.15	3.03	81.82	33
4	Method of randomization	12.12	27.27	60.61	33
5	Blindness of patients to treatment	3.03	3.03	93.94	33
6	Blindness of clinicians to treatment	3.03	0.00	96.97	33
7	Blindness to ongoing results	0.00	0.00	100.00	33
9	Homogeneity check on multicentre data	5.00	15.00	80.00	20
10	Trial size by power calculation	6.06	3.03	90.91	33
11	Other reason for trial size	3.23	0.00	96.77	31
14	Patient reject log	9.09	21.21	69.70	33
16	Exclusion of concomitant diseases	12.12	30.30	57.58	33
18	Identity of comparator in blind studies	0.00	0.00	100.00	2
19	Interruptions to drug administration	7.14	7.14	85.71	28
20	Exclusion of concomitant therapies	9.09	36.36	54.55	33
25	Adverse immunological event reporting	3.03	36.36	60.61	33
26	Uniformity of multicentre evaluations	10.53	15.79	73.68	19
30	Dropout accounting	9.68	35.48	54.84	31
32	Results in terms of trial size	18.75	15.63	65.63	32
Questions which were 'NA' in every case					
21	Length of washout in crossover studies				

*Sample number = the number of trials scored minus the number for which the question was not applicable

the 32 questions for all 33 RCTs of immunotherapy in cancer. Trials of interferon in hairy cell leukaemia are also considered on page 94. Studies on AIDS (Kaposi sarcoma aspects) are also considered in Chapter 6.

Questions which usually scored '2'.

The choice of statistical techniques was generally well done, with life-table analyses and logrank (or similar) tests being used routinely. Several studies had more than two treatment groups, although the statistical features of such designs were not usually mentioned. However, Lessner *et al.* (1984), reporting a trial with four treatment groups, referred to the generalized Kruskal–Wallis method for analysing life-table data (Breslow 1970) as being able to cope with more than two samples (treatment groups). Many accounts simply failed to quote any statistical method at all, even though p values were subsequently reported in the 'Results' section.

Not surprisingly, the questions which deal with such fundamental issues as patient selection, patient numbers, the dosage regimen, and the reporting of results consistently achieved high scores. Even so, there are still lessons to be learned from these questions.

The commonest fault when describing patient selection (question 12) was to give minimal criteria without specifically stating that allcomers were acceptable, thus leaving open to question whether the trialists simply omitted to include the full criteria in the paper.

Most studies reported clearly the numbers of patients enrolled and evaluated per treatment group (question 13). Some, however, gave the number of patients evaluated per group but the number of withdrawals and drop-outs was given only for the trial as a whole, making it impossible to determine how many patients had been lost from each group. As explained in Chapter 4, analysis of withdrawals and drop-outs is essential because there may be a pattern which reflects, for example, lack of efficacy or an unsuspected side-effect or an important practical difficulty influencing drug administration. Giving the number of withdrawals and drop-outs by treatment group is the first stage in such an analysis. Reports of some complex studies would benefit from a flow diagram showing the number of patients evaluated and lost to follow-up at each stage.

Of the four principal features of a dosage regimen—quantity, route, frequency, and duration—the last, duration, was the feature reported least accurately (question 17). Some papers referred to the regimen being administered 'for as long as possible'. This may be meaningful to the trialists but needs qualifying with 'criteria of impossibility' for the final report of the trial.

Clinical methods almost always included CT scans, X-rays, and biopsies where possible. Cell counts were used in studies of haematological malignancies. The studies which scored less than 2 for question '22' generally did so by default because they did not state the monitoring methods in the paper.

Seven of the 33 RCTs included some form of monitoring of immune function. A score of '2' was assigned for studies of responses to tumour specific antigens (Lachmann *et al.* 1985) or NK activity (Groopman *et al.* 1984 and Silver *et al.* 1988). A score of '1' was assigned for monitoring of skin test reactions using antigens related to the trial therapy [e.g. BCG (Omura *et al.* 1982) or tumour cell vaccine (Wunderlich *et al.* 1985)], whilst studies using only standard tests of general immune responsiveness, of no particular relevance to the tumour or the drug, scored '0'.

The reporting of subjective side-effects and reference to laboratory data suggest that side-effects were being actively sought (question 24), although the question used to elicit subjective information from patients was virtually never reported. It should be, however, because the probability of some events being reported will reflect the way in which the enquiry was made.

A common fault in the reporting of the baseline characteristics of the patient groups (question 27) was to state simply that there were no significant differences between the groups in terms of age, sex, or clinical presentation. This needs to be accompanied by a table listing the baseline characteristics of the patients by treatment group, accompanied by the name of the statistical test applied, *p* values and an indication of the range of values observed (e.g. standard deviation, standard error of the mean, confidence intervals, or the range itself). Some trialists performed a multivariate analysis in which the dependence of trial outcome upon baseline characteristics, as well as treatment group, was investigated. Such methods can yield important prognostic information. Some statisticians are of the opinion that such methods should always be applied instead of simply performing numerous Chi-square tests and *t*-tests on baseline data because multiple significance testing should always be avoided under any circumstances. For the purposes of the scoring system used here, however, multivariate analysis was not required in order to score '2'.

Finally, the reporting of results (question 28) usually scored '2'. Occasionally, however, results were published before all of the patients had completed the planned period of follow-up. This could represent the expiry of a deadline for analysis which had been agreed before the start of the trial, in which case there is no danger of bias but the power of the trial is reduced. Alternatively, incomplete follow-up may represent a rush to publish as soon as a result looked interesting. There are various reasons why trialists might feel it necessary to publish early. These include a desire to let the world know about an apparently valuable treatment as soon as possible in order to relieve suffering. Alternatively, there may be pressure to gain another departmental publication in a particular year, or even pressure from a trial sponsor. All of these reasons are unacceptable. A clinical trial is an exercise in probabilities, the value of the result being intimately dependent upon such things as sample size and the elimination of bias. If a horse race could be stopped at any time according to the whim of the punters, then almost any result could be achieved. In the same way, a trial must be left to run its course, although provision can be built into the trial design for sequential or interim analyses which are subject to statistical safeguards against the problems usually associated with multiple looks at the data (Whitehead 1983 and Pocock 1983). Surely it is worse to report an unscheduled and statistically unsound interim result, which might falsely arouse the hopes of patients and doctors, than to wait and publish a reliable result. Early reporting is also disadvantageous to the department or trial sponsors, who may bask temporarily in the glory of the published result only to have to refute it later.

In the occasional paper there was a marked trend towards accentuating the positive results at the expense of the negative ones. Trialists should realize that negative results are important because the complete picture of the properties of a drug includes an account of what it cannot do as well as what it can. Not only is it essential to thus define the limits of the action of a drug, it is unethical for trialists to fail to publish negative results. Other trialists will unwittingly waste the time of patients, and possibly falsely raise their hopes, by administering drugs which have already been shown, elsewhere, to be ineffectual. Such repetitious testing of drugs also wastes the sponsors' money and the valuable time of the trialists, and unnecessarily ties up departmental facilities. It was therefore encouraging that the literature on immunological RCTs included a substantial number of negative reports.

Questions which usually scored '1'.

As discussed above, the most common fault in the reporting of patients numbers (question 13) was to report the number of withdrawals and drop-outs in the trial as a whole rather than by treatment group. Even fewer gave explicit reasons for each withdrawal. Amongst those which did was Gray *et al.* (1989), a study of BCG and tumour cell vaccine in stage B and C large bowel cancer: 'Eight patients were excluded from analysis, six because of stage D disease at the time of trial entry (2 immunotherapy and 4 control group) and two who violated trial protocol by receiving post-operative radio-therapy before disease recurrence had occurred (both immunotherapy group)'. Another example was Silver *et al.* (1988), where the list of non-eligible patients included the statement: 'Eight (3 LDS, 5 HDS) could not tolerate the first course (10 days) of treatment and *as previously specified in the protocol* were evaluable for toxicity, but not response'; ('LDS' and 'HDS' were the treatment groups). Even fewer studies dealt appropriately with the related issue of censorship (question 30) or provided a log of rejected patients (question 14), the usual score being '0' for both (see below).

The reporting of adverse events (question 29) was scanty in many reports, lacking in detail or any indication of the severity or duration of reported events. Kirkwood *et al.* (1985*b*) provide an example of the clear presentation of drug toxicity findings. Each toxic effect was graded for severity and the duration was given. An unfortunate but growing trend in the interferon literature is to refer to the observed adverse event profile as being: 'similar to that observed in other trials of interferon'. Such a statement is meaningless and dangerous. It is meaningless because 'similar' has no absolute comparative value. Events which one trialist would regard as similar, another would regard as very different. It is a dangerous statement because it engenders a lazy attitude towards adverse event reporting with interferon, and raises the question as to how carefully the patients were in fact observed. Is it possible that rare and previously unobserved adverse events could be missed in future trials if such an attitude became common? Questions 16 and 25, also relating to adverse events, usually scored '0' and are discussed below.

Question 31 dealt with the reporting of statistical analyses and usually scored '1' according to the criteria in Chapter 4. Confidence intervals were especially rarely given.

Questions which usually scored '0'.

The majority of the 33 RCTs included in this survey had numerous endpoints. Even when a single endpoint was pursued, the results were often analysed in many different ways. The trialists very rarely indicated which should be regarded as the primary endpoint. The primary endpoint is the one around which the study was designed in terms of patient numbers. Unfortunately, very few studies were designed with statistical power in mind (see below).

The quality of endpoint definition was very variable, with roughly equal numbers of studies scoring '2', '1', and '0'. Endpoints need to be defined unambiguously in order to avoid bias. Most studies which had remission induction as an endpoint included definitions of complete, partial, and minor regression in terms of tumour size or cell counts. Some of these studies, however, failed to report the method used to monitor tumour size. Criteria for relapse were rather less frequently defined. In the same way that partial remission is usually defined in terms of a threshold reduction in tumour size or cell count, so the resumption of growth needs to be defined in terms of a threshold increase in tumour growth or cell count in order to eliminate bias from the judgement of progression. Definition of relapse is especially important when the duration of remission, rather than remission induction, is the primary endpoint of the trial, although some trialists chose not to define relapse in such studies (Golumb *et al.* 1988). In some cases, relapse means the appearance of new tumour following complete disappearance or surgical removal of the primary tumour. It is important here to indicate which of the battery of detection techniques available to the modern clinician will be regarded as giving definitive evidence of a new lesion. Some trialists, for example, required a biopsy of accessible lesions to substantiate X-ray evidence (Lessner *et al.* 1984).

Studies with mortality as an endpoint almost never specified whether or not a particular cause of death should be proven for inclusion in the analysis, although an occasional study listed patients who were excluded because of death from unrelated causes. Trialists should specify whether or not the intention is to analyse all deaths, or to include only particular causes which are relevant to the disease and drug in question. In the latter case, the criteria for establishing cause of death should be given in the form of an endpoint definition.

The importance of obtaining informed consent before randomization was explained in Chapter 4. Most studies failed to mention this point and hence scored '0'. Exceptions include Silver *et al.* (1988), Lessner *et al.* (1984), and Kirkwood *et al.* (1985b), where it is indicated that informed consent was obtained prior to randomization.

The method of randomization was rarely reported, although a brief account would lend credibility to the prerequisite that randomization be performed blind. In one study, a sophisticated procedure (Pocock and Simon 1975) was used to ensure equable distribution of prognostic factors between the treatment groups (Wunderlich *et al.* 1985).

Virtually none of the trials were conducted blind (questions 5, 6, and 7). In one study, oral Levamisole or placebo were administered to ovarian cancer patients in addition to a standard regimen of chemotherapy and radio-therapy (Khoo *et al.* 1984). Apparently, only one patient declined to participate in the study, giving the reason that it involved an experimental drug. In another study of Levamisole, patients randomized to receive active drug did so both pre- and post-operatively, whilst patients randomized to the control group received a placebo for the preoperative part of the trial only (Fox *et al.* 1980). In neither case was the identity of the placebo and active drug mentioned, and hence both studies scored '0' for question 18.

There were 20 multicentre studies amongst the 33 RCTs surveyed. One trial involved no less than 16 collaborating institutions (Ota *et al.* 1986), although only 101 evaluable patients were enrolled among them. It follows that, on average, each centre contributed about three patients to each treatment group during the two and a half years that the study was enrolling patients. Clearly there is considerable scope for variability of patient management and monitoring in such a study, and this variability may well influence the attainment or judgement of treatment success or failure. The 'random noise' thus generated will reduce the clarity of the 'signal', this being defined as the differential efficacy of test and control regimens. Put another way, the statistical power of the study as a whole will be reduced. A further problem of multicentre trials is the interpretation of results when the data from one centre are very different from the data obtained at the other centres, especially if the eccentric result has a strong influence on the overall result.

Questions 9 and 26 refer to two important means of addressing the above problems. The first is to include provision for testing the homogeneity of the data. This could involve simply tabulating the results by centre and checking that the centres are contributing roughly equally, or it could involve including the hospitals as potential prognostic indicators in a multivariate analysis of the trial outcome (Davis *et al.* 1982). Most studies did not address the question of data homogeneity, although some listed the number of patients enrolled by institution. Few reports included reference to the standardization of clinical and laboratory assessments, although some notable exceptions stand out amongst the 33 RCTs surveyed. Hayat *et al.* (1986) was a major international trial involving 23 hospitals in Belgium, France, The Netherlands, and West Germany. The diagnosis of acute myelogenous leukaemia was established for all patients by examination of blood and bone marrow at the World Health Organisation reference centre at Villejuif. An American study on hairy cell leukaemia (Golumb *et al.* 1988) recruited 90 patients from centres in Boston, Buffalo, Chicago, Los Angeles, New Haven, New York, and Seattle but all bone marrow biopsies and blood smears were evaluated by two haematopathologists, one based in Chicago and the other in Duarte (CA). An extra level of objectivity was added by the latter haematopathologist being independent of the trial and not responsible for recruitment of patients.

The most significant flaw detected in the design of RCTs of immunological therapy for cancer was the extraordinarily infrequent use of statistical power calculations to determine the size of studies. Of the 33 RCTs surveyed, only three made some attempt at determining the size of the study in this way. Regarding alternative reasons for the size of the trial sample, Kirkwood *et al.* (1985*b*) conceded that formal proof of superiority of high dose over low dose interferon had been abandoned because the number of patients required greatly exceeded the capacity of the collaborating institutions and the available supplies of interferon. For the other studies, it would have been comforting to know that some objective criterion, such as a predetermined enrolment duration of 5 years, had been used. Otherwise, the scope for bias in these open clinical studies is enormous. One trial included a stopping rule as well as a power calculation (Schiller *et al.* 1989): 'the trial was to be terminated unless five or more responses were observed in the first 14 patients evaluated in the combination (chemotherapy and interferon) arm'.

Of the 20 'high-score' or 'grey-area' RCTs, no less than 14 had no power calculation performed at the outset and ultimately showed no difference between active and control treatments, in terms of efficacy. In an attempt to probe the scope for type II statistical error (the probability of concluding that two treatments have the same efficacy when there is really a difference), power calculations were performed for 22 endpoints amongst these 14 trials according to the method described in Chapter 4. The outcome, which is subject to the limitations discussed in Chapter 4, is shown in Table 5.2. It is apparent that the statistical power of five of the endpoints was less than 80 per cent, even for a test drug outcome of 100 per cent success! Only two endpoints had 80 per cent power to detect a differential between test and control of less than 20 per cent, whilst eight endpoints had 80 per cent power to detect a differential between test and control of 20 to 29 per cent and a further three endpoints had 80 per cent power to detect a differential between test and control of 30 to 39 per cent. Four endpoints had 80 per cent power for differentials above 40 per cent which is expecting rather a lot of the test drug. It follows that, for many of these 22 endpoints, there was a substantial chance of missing a moderately-sized benefit for the test drug.

Several trialists acknowledged their studies were small and the results therefore needed to be proven in larger studies (question 32). Very few, however, performed a formal *post-hoc* power calculation. An example was Lessner *et al.* (1984), in which the size of the trial had

Test drug	Control group	Smallest patient group	% success in control group	Measure of success	% test drug success for 80% power	Test-control differential for 80% power	Reference
aIFN	MELPH+PRED	54	44	RI	70	26	Ahre et al. (1984)
aIFN	NONE	54	60	SVL at 1 yr	84	24	,, (1988)
aIFN HD	aIFN LD	28	69	no relapse post-IFN	96	27	Golumb et al. (1984)
aIFN HD	aIFN LD	10	30	RI	83	53	Groopman et al. (1985)
aIFN HD	aIFN LD	14	7	RI	50	43	Kirkwood et al. (1982)
BCG	CH/NONE	30	0	DF at 4 yrs	21	21	Omura et al. (1982)
		30	8	SVL at 4 yrs	37	29	,,
CPARV+CH	CH	35	26	RI	58	32	Vogl et al. (1985)
CPARV	NONE	80	50	DFS at 3 yrs	72	22	Neifeld et al. (1985)
CPARV	NONE	24	21	SVL at 6 yrs	58	37	Woodruff and Walbaum (1983)
CPARV	T CYCLINE	16	69	RF at 1 month	impossible	–	Leahy et al. (1985)
TCV	CH/NONE	57	70	DF at 2.5 yrs	91	21	Wunderlich et al. (1985)
		57	75	SVL at 2.5 yrs	94	19	,,
BCG+TCV	NONE	7	50	SVL at 3 yrs	impossible	–	Lachmann et al. (1985)
BCG+CH	CH	37	72	DF at 5 yrs	96	24	Giuliano et al. (1986)
BCG+CH+TCV		37	86	SVL at 5 yrs	impossible	–	,,
LEVA+CH	CH	14	50	DFS at 8 yrs	93	43	Sertoli et al. (1987)
		14	49	SVL at 8 yrs	92	43	,,
LEVA+CH	PBO+CH	69	72	RI	91	19	Khoo et al. (1984)
		20	91	SVL at 4 yrs—stage 1	impossible	–	,,
		13	78	SVL at 4 yrs—stage 2	impossible	–	,,
		33	15	SVL at 4 yrs—stage 3	45	30	,,

Key:
DF   = Disease free
DFS = Disease free survival
RI   = Response incidence
SVL = Survival
Other abbreviations as in Appendices (p. 113)

been determined by a statistical power calculation but unfortunately the estimated incidence of recurrence and death used in the calculation proved to be overestimates. This resulted in a drastically reduced statistical power, estimated by the trialists to be only 60 per cent for the detection of a 50 per cent difference in efficacy between treatments. There was thus a 40 per cent chance of having failed to observe a very large difference between treatments. It follows that the chance of detecting a smaller, more realistic difference was very low indeed.

Comments about adverse immunological events (question 25) were limited to the transient reduction of cell counts accompanying interferon or levamisole and the local reactions associated with the use of agents such as BCG.

Dropout accounting (question 30) was generally poorly done according to the criteria in Chapter 4. However, some studies did indicate the level of censorship on the Kaplan–Meier plots (e.g. Maver *et al.* 1982). Others noted the total number censored per group over the whole time period of the trial (e.g. Vogler *et al.* 1984). Some reports indicated that all patients had been followed up for a specified period of time, such as Ochiai *et al.* (1983), in which all surviving patients had attained at least 3 years' participation.

Very few trials included a reject log (question 14), sufficient information about the exclusion of concomitant disease (question 16) or drugs (question 20) or information about interruptions to treatment administration (question 19). These questions usually scored '0' according to the criteria in Chapter 4.

QC check

The 20 studies which scored at least 34 per cent overall ('grey-area' and 'high-score' studies) were subjected to four further questions concerning quality control of the trial as explained in Chapter 4. The questions related to the auditing of case report forms and, where appropriate, to tests of blindness, compliance for self-administered regimens and checks for any effects of sample transportation upon the reliability of laboratory data in multicentre studies. None of these QC measures were employed by any of the 33 RCTs surveyed.

NRCTs

The NRCT scores ranged from 33 per cent to 87 per cent with a median of 56 per cent and a mean of 57 per cent. There was no evidence for the quality of the trials improving with time. The scores achieved by the NRCTs were tested for correlation with year of publication and none was found ($R^2 = 0.147$). Trials of interferon in hairy cell leukaemia are also considered on page 94. Studies on AIDS (Kaposi sarcoma aspects) are also considered in Chapter 6.

This section covers some especially novel and intriguing approaches to the treatment of cancer, including trials with LAK cells (the patient's own lymphocytes activated *ex vivo* by lymphokines and re-infused), radiolabelled antibodies ('targeted radiotherapy') and anti-idiotypes. Colony Stimulating Factors (CSF) are under investigation as part of a strategy to avoid the myelosuppression associated with cancer chemotherapy. Brandt *et al.* (1988) removed a sample of the patient's bone marrow before chemotherapy was commenced and re-implanted it afterwards, CSF being used to accelerate bone marrow re-establishment. In terms of trial methodology, one of the most important studies in this survey was that of Bernengo *et al.* (1983) on melanoma. Stage 1 patients were enrolled only if they had a demonstrable T cell deficiency, previous work having established that such patients have a lower probability of survival and that a fall in T cell numbers usually accompanied or preceded recurrence. This work clearly provided a rationale for using an immunomodulator, unlike so many trials in which no evidence of immunodeficiency is available and immunomodulators are used merely on the presumption of an immunodeficiency permitting survival of the tumour.

As shown in Table 5.3, the outcome of scoring the NRCTs was remarkably similar to the outcome for the RCTs. All of the questions which scored '2' in the RCT scheme did so in the NRCT scheme except for 'choice of statistical methods' (question 6 in the NRCT scheme and 8 in the RCT scheme). However, even for this question there was a remarkable underlying similarity. In both cases, methods were chosen well (score '2') or badly (score '0') with very few mediocre choices (score '1'). Also in both cases, the proportion of trials scoring '2' was very close to that scoring '0'.

The questions dealing with patient withdrawals and drop-out accounting scored better for NRCTs than for RCTs, reflecting the more detailed reporting which is possible for the smaller series of patients recruited into NRCTs. Adverse events were reported more fully for NRCTs reflecting the preoccupation of early-phase clinical trials with toxicity. A smaller proportion of NRCTs than RCTs were multicentre studies (32 per cent and 61 per cent respectively). Whereas all of the RCTs involved statistical testing, only 38 per cent of NRCTs did so. Oberg *et al.* (1983) provide an example of a study in which the authors tested the data for normal distribution before applying a *t*-test. Logarithmic transformation was used to render the data distribution normal

Table 5.3 Score frequencies for each question (NRCTs)

Question number	Subject of question	Score frequency (per cent)			Sample* number
		2	1	0	
Questions which usually scored '2'					
2	Definition of endpoints	61.70	14.89	23.40	47
9	Reporting of patient selection criteria	78.72	21.28	0.00	47
10	Reporting of patient numbers	87.23	12.77	0.00	47
12	Patient withdrawal log	79.17	12.50	8.33	24
14	Reporting of dosage regimen	78.72	21.28	0.00	47
18	Length of washout in crossover studies	66.67	0.00	33.33	3
19	Objectivity of clinical monitoring	80.85	8.51	10.64	47
20	Relevance of immunological monitoring	68.75	6.25	25.00	16
21	Close monitoring for adverse events	65.96	29.79	4.26	47
24	Reporting of baseline patient data	80.85	14.89	4.26	47
25	Reporting of results	63.83	34.04	2.13	47
26	Adverse event reporting	59.57	40.43	0.00	47
27	Dropout accounting	35.00	35.00	30.00	20
Questions which usually scored '1'					
22	Adverse immunological event reporting	10.64	51.06	38.30	47
Questions which usually scored '0'					
1	Number of endpoints	0.00	0.00	100.00	7
3	Blindness of patients to treatment	0.00	0.00	100.00	4
4	Blindness of clinicians to treatment	0.00	0.00	100.00	4
5	Blindness to ongoing results	0.00	0.00	100.00	4
6	Choice of statistical methods	38.89	16.67	44.44	18
7	Homogeneity check on multicentre data	0.00	6.67	93.33	15
8	Reason for trial size	2.13	2.13	95.74	47
11	Patient reject log	6.38	0.00	93.62	47
13	Exclusion of concomitant diseases	23.40	19.15	57.45	47
16	Interruptions to drug administration	10.87	30.43	58.70	46
17	Exclusion of concomitant therapies	10.64	38.30	51.06	47
23	Uniformity of multicentre evaluations	8.33	8.33	83.33	12
28	Statistical reporting	16.67	38.89	44.44	18
Questions which were 'NA' in every case					
15	Identity of comparator in blind studies				

*Sample number = the number of trials scored minus the number for which the question was not applicable

if necessary. Statistical reporting most frequently scored '0' for NRCTs and '1' for RCTs. However, in both cases, the score distribution was very similar (i.e. 48.48 per cent scored '1' and 42.42 per cent scored '0' for RCTs; 38.89 per cent scored '1' and 44.44 percent scored '0' for NRCTs), indicating a similar trend for NRCTs and RCTs.

Early phase clinical trials are usually exploratory and therefore have numerous endpoints. For this reason, question 1, referring to the number of endpoints was rated 'NA' for all non-comparative trials. There were only seven comparative NRCTs, including studies with historical controls (Brandt *et al*. 1988 and Nemunaitis *et al*. 1988), alternate treatment designs (Antman *et al*. 1988 and Gabrilove *et al*. 1988) and non-randomized concurrent controls (Bernengo *et al*. 1983). All of these had two or more endpoints or strata. Curiously, the endpoints for NRCTs were usually defined, which was not the case for RCTs (question 2). A frequent principal NRCT endpoint was induction of remission, whereas the endpoint for RCTs was usually incidence of relapse. As has been noted already, whilst trialists usually define the former they rarely define the latter.

The use of historical controls is controversial. For example, Lessner *et al*. (1984) concluded that the result obtained from comparison with a randomized control group was quite different from the result which would have been obtained with a historical control group. In the randomized comparison of BCG extract with chemotherapy as adjuvant to surgery for colon cancer, the overall survival in both treatment groups was far better than previously seen in this indication. No advantage was observed for the BCG group in the randomized study. Had the BCG result been compared only with historical data, then the conclusion would have been drawn that BCG was effective for, in this case, spurious reasons.

All but one NRCT lacked any indication of why the stated number of patients had been enrolled, thus providing a source of bias. As discussed in Chapter 4, it is essential that the size of the patient sample be determined by some objective means in order to avoid the publication of results when they are looking good, rather than when a firm result has been obtained. The analogy of a horse race was drawn, in which almost any result could be obtained if the punters could choose to stop the trial at any time. For an NRCT, there are various criteria for deciding the size of a trial, including the agreement to enrol all presenting patients over a fixed period of time or the sample size required for a valid statistical comparison with the null hypothesis. The latter method was used by the only trial to quote a reason for the trial size (Creagan *et al*. 1988), in which the ability of aspirin to reduce the side-effects of interferon was investigated. A premature stopping rule for the trial was built into these statistical considerations, thus illustrating the applicability of such methods to NRCTs.

Immunological monitoring usually scored '2', investigation of NK cytotoxicity being common amongst the 16 studies which monitored immune function. Three studies investigated *in vitro* cytotoxicity to fresh tumour samples (Fischer *et al*. 1988; Lotze *et al*. 1986 and Yoshida *et al*. 1988). One study (Lotze *et al*. 1986) included tests for IL-2 receptor mRNA expression using a DNA hybridization technique.

Adverse immunological events were commented upon somewhat more frequently than for the RCTs, but this reflects the larger proportion of interferon studies in the sample of NRCTs. Monitoring of cell numbers in interferon studies is routine because of the commonly observed transient myelosuppression. Other events included graft rejection (Jacobs *et al*. 1985), joint inflammation (Quesada *et al*. 1986*a*), and autoimmune phenomena (Eriksson *et al*. 1986; Oberg *et al*. 1986).

The same range of QC questions was applied to NRCTs which scored at least 50 per cent as was applied to RCTs which achieved at least 34 per cent. Again, none referred to auditing of case report forms, although one (Merchant *et al*. 1988) stated that the trial had been conducted according to FDA guidelines and therefore presumably involved auditing. Of the studies which involved self-administration, or administration by a family member, only one reported compliance information (Creagan *et al*. 1988). This study required the patients to take aspirin four times daily whilst interferon was administered by the trialists. Data were reported for the aspirin regimen and the results provide a guide to the level of compliance which can be expected, even of highly motivated cancer patients. Less than half of the patients (41 per cent) took at least 90 per cent of the required regimen whilst 7 per cent of the patients took less than 50 per cent. These data suggest that compliance with self-administered injection of interferon, as opposed to oral administration of aspirin, should be carefully investigated. No other QC measures were reported in these studies.

Trials of interferon in hairy cell leukaemia

Efficacy

The greatest success yet achieved with an immunological substance as a treatment for cancer is the use of alpha-interferon for hairy cell leukaemia (HCL). This chronic leukaemia of unknown aetiology is rare (<2 per cent of all leukaemias) and is characterized by the presence of a unique type of cell in peripheral blood and bone marrow. These 'hairy cells' have a distinctive morphology and, often, the unusual combination of cell-surface immunoglobulin and interleukin-2 (IL-2) receptors. Whilst they do not have C3 receptors, distinguishing them from monocytes, they are capable of phagocytosis. Despite the presence of IL-2 receptors, suggesting a T-lymphocyte origin, they do not form rosettes with sheep red blood cells. The disease affects roughly four times as many men as women, and is characterized by neutropaenia, thrombocytopaenia, and anaemia resulting in repeated infection and weakness. Typical survival is 3–5 years, although some patients survive much longer. Early death is usually due to overwhelming infection.

Of the clinical studies surveyed, 2 'high-score' NRCTs, 3 'grey-area' NRCTs, 1 'low-score' NRCT and 1 'grey-area' RCT involved the treatment of HCL with alpha-interferon. The NRCTs concerned the induction of remission as a primary endpoint, whilst the RCT addressed the question of the duration of remission after cessation of interferon administration. Table 5.4(a) summarizes the data on remission induction obtained with the 153 evaluable patients in the six 'high-score' and 'grey-area' studies. It is apparent that a very high level of response was obtained, comprising 18 per cent complete and 68 per cent partial responses. No less than 92 per cent of patients showed some degree of response.

The seminal study was that of Quesada *et al.* (1984), in which 7 patients received 3×10^6 units of a partially purified alpha-interferon daily by the intramuscular route. Five patients had failed previous treatments [splenectomy (5), chemotherapy (2) and BCG extract (1)], whilst two had not previously been treated but had evidence of progressive disease. The criteria for response were very well defined, complete remission being defined as the attainment of *all* the following criteria: no hairy cells in the bone marrow aspirate and biopsy, bone marrow granulocytes above 35 per cent, a normal distribution of cell membrane markers of bone marrow mononuclear cells, haemoglobin at least 12 g/dl, absolute neutrophil count at least 1500 cells/mm^3, platelet count at least 10^5/mm^3. This is an excellent example of a single endpoint being derived from the monitoring of several variables, thus avoiding the need for mutiple significance testing and greatly increasing the ease with which the reader can assimilate the trial outcome. A similarly detailed definition of partial remission was also given. All seven patients in this initial trial responded to interferon therapy, there being three complete and four partial remissions. These overall results were supported by tables of individual patient data.

The use of a partially purified interferon preparation raised the

Table 5.4(a) Efficacy of aIFN in hairy cell leukaemia: induction of remission

Trial	Patients enrolled	Patients evaluable	Complete responses	(per cent)	Partial responses	(per cent)	Minor responses	(per cent)	Duration of therapy at time result reported
Thompson *et al.* (1985)	14	13	3	23.1	10	76.9	ND	—	complete = 6–10 months partial = approx. 3 months
Quesada *et al.* (1984)	7	7	3	42.9	4	57.1	ND	—	6–10 months
Quesada *et al.* (1986*a*)	30	30	9	30.0	17	56.7	ND	—	not clear
Golumb *et al.* (1988)*	90	81	12	14.8	62	76.5	7	8.6	12 months
Ratain *et al.* (1985)	9	8	0	0.0	5	62.5	3	37.5	44–52 weeks
Jacobs *et al.* (1985)	22	14	0	0.0	6	42.9	ND	—	6 months
Totals	172	153	27	17.6	104	68.0	10	6.5	

* Result taken from the initial phase of the trial in which all patients received Interferon for remission induction prior to randomization in a study of remission duration.

question of whether or not the therapeutic activity resided in the interferon or in an impurity. The subsequent five studies listed in Table 5.4(a) all used recombinant alpha-interferons and the high level of efficacy obtained indicates that interferon, rather than any impurity, is indeed responsible for the observed remission of HCL.

All of these results are very encouraging. However, there remains considerable variation in response rates amongst trials of interferon in this indication, and this was observed in the sample of six trials included here. The incidence of complete response ranged from 0 per cent to 42.9 per cent, whilst a partial response was observed in 42.9–76.9 per cent of patients. Some insight into this variation can be gained by comparing trial design features such as patient selection and dosage regimen. As shown on pages 81 and 92, these features were usually well reported and indeed they have been discussed as possible reasons for the different results obtained with interferon in this indication (Quesada *et al.* 1986*a*). It has also been suggested that the variation in results might follow from recording remissions after different periods of follow-up, although this does not appear to be the case in the sample of studies included here (Table 5.4(a)). Whilst differences in patient selection or dosage regimen may indeed be the reasons for variation in the results, and it is important to remember that an effective drug will show a dose-response relationship, we draw attention here to some of the methodological sources of variation between studies that could also be responsible for variation in the results.

Table 5.4(b) lists some methodological comparisons between these studies. The information comes from questions 2, 16, 19, and 20 of the scoring system for RCTs and 2, 13, 16, and 17 of the scoring system for NRCTs as well as QC question (iii). All of these questions usually scored '0' (or 'no' in the case of the QC question), with the exception of question 2 in the NRCT scheme, and it is clear that without more definitive statements direct comparison of the trials is difficult.

Firstly, when the incidence of remission in these studies is compared, it is clear that the definitions of the endpoints are not uniform. In fact, as Table 5.4(b) shows, only two of six trials have identical definitions of complete remission and none have identical definitions of partial or minor responses. Yet some published reviews provide tables of cumulative data unqualified by comments as to the similarity or otherwise of response criteria. In the sample of six trials considered here, the definitions of complete response are similar but the definitions of partial response are quite different. Amongst the definitions of complete response, the difference between endpoints 'A' and 'B' raises questions about the sensitivity of the monitoring technique, whilst endpoint 'K' will correlate

Table 5.4(b) Methodological features of trials of aIFN in hairy cell leukaemia

Trial	Minimum regimen specified for inclusion in analysis?	Interruptions to regimen reported?	Self-administration of drug by patient?	Compliance testing?	Concomitant diseases excluded?	Concomitant medication excluded?	Definition of endpoints (CR= complete response, PR=partial response, MR= minor response)
Thompson et al. (1985)	not specified	no	yes	no	no	no	CR: A and D and H and K PR: F or I
Quesada et al. (1984)	not specified	1 'temporary discontinuation' due to adverse event	no	—	no	no	CR: A and G and H and J PR: C and G and H
Quesada et al. (1986a)	not specified	no	no	—	no	no	CR: A and D and H PR: C* and H
Golumb et al. (1988)	patients judged after 12 months of treatment	no	yes	no	some	'preferably' no treatment in past 4 weeks	CR: B and H PR: H +/− C MR: I
Ratain et al. (1985)	'patients evaluated after a minimum of 8 weeks after beginning IFN therapy'	no	yes	no	some	'preferably' no treatment in past 4 weeks	CR: A and H PR: D and H MR: E or I

Jacobs *et al.* (1985)	8 weeks	'no patient required discontinuation due to symptomatic side-effects'; 1 patient stopped for one week due to rejection of a corneal transplant	yes	no	no	all treatments discontinued at least 1 month before	CR: B and H PR: C

Key:

A = HC in BM = 0
B = HC in BM to <5 per cent absolute
C = HC in BM to <50 per cent of baseline
C* = (per cent cellularity × per cent HC) in BM to <50 per cent of baseline
D = HC in PB = 0
E = HC in PB to <5 per cent absolute
F = HC in BM or PB to <10 per cent of baseline
G = BM granulocytes >35 per cent absolute
H = all of: Hb >12 g/dl; neutrophils >1500/mm^3; platelets >100,000/mm^3
I = one of: Hb >12 g/dl; neutrophils >1500/mm^3; platelets >100,000/mm^3 (precise thresholds altered in some studies)
J = normal distribution of BM mononuclear markers
K = absence of transfusion requirement

BM = bone marrow
PB = peripheral blood

Table 5.5(a) Adverse events encountered during the use of aIFN in hairy cell leukaemia

	Thompson et al. (1985)	Quesada et al. (1984)	Quesada et al. (1986a)	Ratain et al. (1985)	Jacobs et al. (1985)
Enrolled patients:	14	7	30	9	22
Evaluable patients:	13	7	30	8	14
Events:					
abnormal taste				2	
alopecia				1	
anorexia		6			
apathy					
arthralgia	yes	1			
asthenia		1			
changed LFTs	6				
decreased libido					
dry mouth			10		
fatigue	yes	7	'most'	5	'common'
fever	yes		'most'	7	22
gonadal failure	3			8	
gynecomastia	3				
headache	yes			3	
hepatitis				4	
'influenza'	yes	yes		5	
myalgia	yes			2	'common'
paresthesia					
weight loss		no			
death on therapy				1	1
adverse immune events:					
transient myelosuppression			some	yes	yes
other			3		1

Table 5.5(b) Further methodological features of trials of aIFN in hairy cell leukaemia

Trial	Concomitant diseases excluded?	Concomitant medication excluded?	Close monitoring: subjective events and biochem. tests?	Adverse immune events	Adverse event reporting: severity and duration given?
Thompson *et al.* (1985)	no	no	yes	no	some
Quesada *et al.* (1984)	no	no	yes	no	yes
Quesada *et al.* (1986*a*)	no	no	no biochem. tests	yes	yes
Ratain *et al.* (1985)	some	'preferably' no treatment in past 4 weeks	yes	yes	some
Jacobs *et al.* (1985)	no	all treatments discontinued at least 1 month before	yes	yes	yes

with endpoint 'H' and may not provide a greater hurdle to be crossed by the patients. Amongst the definitions of partial response, some require all three cytopaenias to be corrected (Quesada *et al.* 1984, 1986a; Golumb *et al.* 1988; and Ratain *et al.* 1985), whilst one requires that only one cytopaenia be corrected (Thompson *et al.* 1985) and one considers only the bone marrow response (Jacobs *et al.* 1985). (The latter study considered the response of the cytopaenias as separate endpoints.) The degree of reduction of hairy cell count, in bone marrow and/or peripheral blood, required for a partial response also differed between the studies: at least 50 per cent reduction of hairy cells in bone marrow (Quesada *et al.* 1984 and Jacobs *et al.* 1985); at least 50 per cent reduction in leukaemic infiltrate of bone marrow, defined as cellularity times per cent hairy cells (Quesada *et al.* 1986a); absence of hairy cells in peripheral blood (Ratain *et al.* 1985); at least 90 per cent reduction of hairy cells in bone marrow *or* peripheral blood (Thompson *et al.* 1985). Golumb *et al.* (1988) defined two forms of partial response depending upon whether or not the bone marrow hairy cell count was reduced. These two forms of partial response were not, however, distinguished in the reported results. The definition of partial response for Thompson *et al.* (1985) would include patients who were regarded only as minor responders in Ratain *et al.* (1985) and Golumb *et al.* (1988). Of these three papers, only Ratain *et al.* (1985) provide individual patient data, thus allowing re-evaluation of the results according to the criteria of another study. If evaluated according to the criteria of Thompson *et al.* (1985), the study with the highest reported incidence of partial remission, then there were no less than six partial remissions at 9–30 weeks in Ratain *et al.* (1985) rather than the two reported by the authors. The importance of defining endpoints is thus clear.

Very little information was given to indicate that the proposed dosage regimen was adhered to. Only one study clearly defined a minimum period of interferon administration to qualify for evaluation (Jacobs *et al.* 1985). Four studies did not indicate whether or not there had been any gaps in administration. Most importantly, four of the trials required the patients to administer the interferon themselves and yet no compliance testing, such as ampoule accounting, was reported. Surely this is especially relevant when the treatment is administered by injection rather than by the oral route, and even more relevant when the treatment induces clear side-effects. Amongst the adverse events encountered in some cases were: fatigue, apathy, pain, and loss of libido (see Table 5.5(a)). Do we know that all of these patients really received the interferon at all? Presumably this information was provided in the case report forms supplied to the regulatory authorities in order to permit the granting of a product licence for interferon in this indication. Curiously, the only report which did mention compliance did not involve self-administration (Quesada *et al.* 1986*a*).

It was not the intention of this analysis to attempt to seek correlations in so small a sample of studies, but rather to provide a methodological critique. It is apparent, however, that the two trials with the highest incidence of complete remission (Quesada *et al.* 1984, 1986*a*) did not involve self-administration. Such a suggestion could be investigated in further trials. If substantiated, then the company that will corner the market for interferon in this indication will be the one which develops a simple and quick method of administration that encourages compliance, such as a box of spring-loaded, single-use syringe devices which already contain the requisite dosage.

Of course, none of this is intended to decry the value of 'intention-to-treat' trials. It may well be that the trialists wished to test interferon in this indication under the rigours of self-administration. The true aim of the trial may have been to determine not just the incidence of remission but, instead, the incidence of remission when some injections are missed. Such a study could be an important indicator of the true value of a drug in everyday use. It would be helpful, however, if the trialists would indicate this in the paper.

Another confounding factor to the success of a clinical trial is the administration of concomitant medications which influence the attainment of trial endpoints or interfere with the immune system. Only two of the trials in Table 5.4(b) excluded patients with (some) serious diseases and none unequivocally excluded concomitant medication. It follows that patients could have been receiving treatment for another indication which was interfering with the trial therapy. The unknown level of concomitant medication provides another potential source of variation between the studies which could be reflected in the responses obtained.

The primary aim of Golumb *et al.* (1988) was to investigate the duration of remission after cessation of interferon administration. Eighty-one evaluable patients received interferon therapy for 1 year. They were then randomized to receive either a further 6 months' interferon or no further interferon. The incidence of relapse and the level of cytopaenia were monitored from the time of cessation of interferon (at 12 months in one group and 18 months in the other) and were shown to be similar. The authors therefore conclude there to be no benefit, post-treatment, to be derived from a longer initial period of interferon administration. Unfortunately, the authors did not provide a definition of the recurrence endpoint, leaving the judgement to the discretion of the individual investigators in this multicentre study, even though they had very carefully defined complete and partial remission in terms of cell counts. In this instance, however, remission was not a trial endpoint but, rather, a patient selection criterion. It is especially important to define recurrence when, as in this case, patients with only partial remission are followed up for relapse. Whereas relapse from complete remission involves, in most studies, the reappearance of hairy cells from a baseline of zero and is easily and unequivocally determined, relapse from partial remission is more complicated. It involves an increase in the number of hairy cells, the magnitude of which varies between patients. Further, the baseline against which each increase is judged will vary between patients. Each trialists' assessment of recurrence will vary unless a threshold percentage increase is specified above which the patient is considered to have relapsed. This is strictly analogous to defining partial remission as a threshold percentage reduction in the hairy cell count.

Safety

Table 5.5(a) lists the adverse events reported in the five 'high-score' or 'grey-area' trials dealing with remission induction. (The report of adverse events in Golumb *et al.* (1988) concerns only those observed after 1 year of interferon therapy, and is considered below.) Several reporting styles are apparent, ranging from the numerical incidence (the most useful), through the descriptive (i.e. 'most' or 'common') to comments which give no indication of frequency (i.e. 'yes') which are the least useful.

It is apparent that fever, myalgia, and fatigue, sometimes described as an influenza-like syndrome, usually accompany interferon administration. These symptoms can arise within hours of commencing interferon (Jacobs *et al.* 1985) but usually fade away with continued interferon administration (Ratain *et al.* 1985 and Thompson *et al.* 1985). The severity of fever is dose related (Ratain *et al.* 1985 and Quesada *et al.* 1986*a*) and sometimes severe enough to warrant hospitalization (Ratain *et al.* 1985). Whilst infection is not uncommon in HCL, overt infection does not appear to correlate with the onset or duration of the influenza-like symptoms. In one study, for example, only 2 of 22 patients developed overt infection (one lobar pneumonia and one *Staphylococcus aureus*), although all patients experienced fever (Jacobs *et al.* 1985). One report confirmed that fever, myalgia, and headache were not present before commencement of interferon (Thompson *et al.* 1985).

A diverse range of further adverse events was reported from the above trials and the elucidation of their true relevance to interferon therapy must await the accumulation of data on far more patients. Few patients were withdrawn from the trials because of adverse events, the usual strategy being to reduce the dosage until their severity became tolerable. As noted above, the nature of some of the symptoms suggests that compliance should be monitored carefully when patients administer the regimen themselves.

The two deaths on therapy both occurred during the first week of interferon therapy in patients with thrombocytopaenia, and were due to cerebral accident (Jacobs *et al.* 1985) and intracerebral haemorrhage (Ratain *et al.* 1985). The extent to which these events could be related to interferon therapy, in the light of the initial myelosuppression outlined below, was not discussed by the authors. However, Ratain *et al.* (1985) reported that no patient required platelet transfusion and no mention is made of platelet administration by Jacobs *et al.* (1985), although red cell transfusions are reported. It therefore appears that the platelet counts in these two patients did not fall below the threshold indicating transfusion in the days prior to death. It follows that if there is a relationship between these deaths and interferon administration, then it does not involve a simple effect upon the platelet count.

General comments used by the trialists to summarize their experience of the tolerability of interferon were: 'well-tolerated' (Jacobs *et al.* 1985), 'well tolerated in all but one patient' (Quesada *et al.* 1984), 'tolerance . . . excellent' (Quesada *et al.* 1986a), or 'toxicity . . . in all patients' (Ratain *et al.* 1985).

Five questions in the scoring system relate to the detection and reporting of adverse events, *viz.*: questions 16, 20, 24, 25, and 29 in the RCT scheme and 13, 17, 21, 22, and 26 in the NRCT scheme. Table 5.5(b) summarizes the responses to these questions for the five trials which reported on the incidence of adverse events during remission induction.

The lack of a statement regarding the exclusion or non-exclusion of concomitant diseases or treatments confounds any attempt to ascribe all but the most commonly observed events unequivocally to interferon. Similarly, the lack of routine screening for common autoantibodies prevents any comments from being made about the incidence of auto-immune phenomena. Only one study included such a screen (Quesada *et al.* 1986a), and this was performed because of symptoms of joint inflammation rather than as part of routine monitoring.

The detection of adverse events depends upon how hard they are sought. All reports included subjective symptoms as well as objective signs, thus indicating that patients were questiond as well as observed. The question used to elicit this information was not usually reported. As discussed in Chapter 4, it would be helpful if trialists would provide this information because the probability of some events being reported is dependent upon the way the patient is asked about them. Four studies also made some mention of biochemical testing. Both the severity and duration of adverse events were usually reported.

The unwanted immunological effects comprised one case of transplant rejection (Jacobs *et al.* 1985) and three cases of joint inflammation with arthritis and/or vasculitis (Quesada *et al.* 1986*a*). In the former case, a 10-year-old corneal transplant was rejected 2 weeks after commencing interferon. Trial therapy was stopped for 1 week and prednisone administered as eyedrops. The rejection episode ceased and did not recur when interferon was restarted. A causal relationship between the joint inflammation and interferon was considered remote by the trialists, who commented that such disorders complicate the course of HCL in up to 24 per cent of patients. However, none of the other trials of interferon in HCL included in this survey mentioned such events. Two cases resolved spontaneously whilst one required corticosteroids. Transient myelosuppression, manifested as an initial worsening of cytopaenia, was reported in three studies. Jacobs *et al.* (1985) reported a fall in granulocyte, erythrocyte, and platelet count in the first 4 weeks, followed by a steady increase over the subsequent 4 weeks. Initial worsening of cytopaenia was well documented by Ratain *et al.* (1985), who provided data on the magnitude of the decrease (mean and range), the time to nadir (median and range), and the duration (median and range). The trialists report that one patient required transfusion because of their anaemia and two patients were hospitalized for neutropaenic fevers during the first 3 weeks of interferon administration.

Golumb *et al.* (1988) reported that the incidence of fatigue was greater in the extended (18 month) treatment group than in the 12-month group. Influenza-like symptoms were also commonplace. This report, however, contains the statement that 'other toxic effects were similar to those reported previously (data not shown)', the undesirability of which was discussed in detail above. Dermatological and neurological disorders were also reported, but their nature, duration, and severity were not reported. The adverse event profile of patients receiving extended interferon therapy therefore needs to be investigated further.

Mechanism of action of 'high-score' agents

Efficacy was demonstrated in 'high-score' trials for: alpha-interferon, IL-2 +/− LAK, GM-CSF and anti-idiotypes.

Those attempting to unravel the mechanism of action of interferon are spoilt for choice in terms of the wide range of *in vitro* properties which have been demonstrated. The quantitative *in vivo* relevance of any of these effects remains unknown. Quesada (1987) has provided an overview of the possible mechanisms of action of interferon in HCL and the available evidence for each. These include the following:

1. The well established anti-viral properties of interferon could be responsible for efficacy if HCL has a viral aetiology. This is difficult to establish because infection may be secondary to the immunodeficiency associated with HCL rather than a causative factor.

2. Interferon could suppress the expression of oncogenes in the hairy cells. The oncogenes could represent, for example, the over-expression of a normal growth factor receptor gene, the de-repression of a gene coding for an autocrine growth stimulant, the repression of a gene coding for a normal growth inhibitor, or the abnormal expression of a signal transduction component downstream from the interaction between normal growth factor(s) and receptor(s). Any of these could result in the hairy cells escaping from the normal controls on growth and differentiation.

3. The well established immunomodulatory properties of interferon, including the stimulation of NK cell activity by alpha-interferon, could be relevant if there is evidence of defective or reduced immune function (as opposed to cell numbers) in HCL patients. This may be difficult to establish because of the small number of cells available for study.

4. Interferon may modulate the production of growth and differentiation substances which restore the number of immunological cells to a level at which the hairy cells can be eliminated.

5. Interferon may modulate the expression of surface antigens on the hairy cells, rendering them more antigenic.

6. Interferon may overcome a 'maturation block' which has inhibited the final stage(s) of development of the hairy cells into mature lymphocytes. This could take place by direct or indirect means, with interferon itself inducing maturation or facilitating the action of endogenous growth and differentiation signals.

7. Exogenous interferon may simply correct an endogenous deficiency of interferon. Such a deficiency could be responsible for the failure of the hairy cells to achieve maturation.

8. Any combination of the above mechanisms. For example, oncogene expression could be triggered by a virus and interferon could block this process, both by direct inhibition of the virus and an effect upon gene expression. Alternatively, interferon may overcome a 'maturation block' which allows the hairy cells to develop to a stage of differentiation at which they are more susceptible to destruction by the immune system.

Interferons as well as IL-2 and GM-CSF, belong to the large family of cytokines whose role in cancer therapy was reviewed extensively by Balkwill (1988). The physiological roles of IL-2 and GM-CSF, as promoters of events such as cellular proliferation and differentiation, provide an explanation of the mechanism of action of these agents in, for example, the *ex vivo* stimulation of lymphocytes with IL-2 (Rosenberg *et al.* 1987) or acceleration of bone marrow re-establishment with GM-CSF (Brandt *et al.* 1988).

The rationale for using anti-idotypes in cancer therapy (Meeker *et al.* 1985) follows from the belief that most human B-cell malignancies are derived from a single aberrant cell, the resulting clone therefore carrying a unique surface immunoglobulin idiotype. Anti-idiotype antibodies will thus act as exquisitely specific anti-tumour antibodies.

Appendix 5.1: List of randomized cancer trials included in this survey

Test drug	Test patients evaluated	Control group	Control patients evaluated	Form of cancer	Outcome of scoring	Reference
aIFN	26	NONE	31	myeloma	LS	Mandelli et al. (1988)
aIFN	28	NONE	35	Hairy Cell Leukaemia	GA	Golumb et al. (1988)
aIFN	74	MELPH+PRED	54	myeloma	GA	Ahre et al. (1984)
aIFN (HD)	10	aIFN (LD)	10	Kaposi sarcoma	GA	Groopman et al. (1984)
aIFN (HD)	16	aIFN (LD)	14	renal	GA	Kirkwood et al. (1985b)
aIFN (HD)	23	aIFN (LD)	30	breast/ovarian/osteogenic	GA	Silver et al. (1988)
				non-Hodgkin/nasopharyngeal	GA	
bIFN+gIFN+CH	18	CH	18	lung	HS	Schiller et al. (1989)
BCGextr	142	NONE/CH	290	colon	GA	Lessner et al. (1984)
BCGextr+CH	140					
BCG	30	CH/NONE	67	acute myelogenous leukaemia	GA	Omura et al. (1982)
BCG+CH	111	CH	127	breast	LS	Buzdar et al. (1984)
BCG+CH	51	CH	51	acute myelogenous leukaemia	LS	Vogler et al. (1984)
BCG	56					
BCGextr+CH	49	NONE/CH	89	gastric	GA	Ochiai et al. (1983)
BCG+CH	51	CH	66	lung	LS	Maver et al. (1982)
BCG+CH+H	100	CH+/−H	200	breast	LS	Hubay et al. (1985)
NOCextr	52	NONE	64	lung	GA	Yasumoto et al. (1985)
NOCextr+CH	115	CH	98	gastric	GA	Koyama et al. (1986)
CPARV	15	T'CYCLINE	13	lung (pleural effusions)	GA	Leahy et al. (1985)
CPARV	25	NONE	24	lung	GA	Woodruff and Walbaum et al. (1983)
CPARV	96	NONE	80	oral/pharyngeal/laryngeal	GA	Neifeld et al. (1985)
CPARV	44	NONE?	48	colorectal	LS	Souter et al. (1982)
CPARV+CH	38	CH	35	head and neck	GA	Vogl et al. (1982)
PROPI+CH	38	CH	41	lung	LS	Roszkowski et al. (1985)
TCV	57	CH/NONE	121	colorectal	GA	Wunderlich et al. (1985)
TCV+CH	28	CH+/−H*	105	acute myelogenous leukaemia	GA	Hayat et al. (1986)

Appendix 5.1: *(cont)*

Test drug	Test patients evaluated	Control group	Control patients evaluated	Form of cancer	Outcome of scoring	Reference
BCG+CH	53	CH	37	breast	GA	Giuliano et al. (1986)
BCG+CH+TCV	41					
BCG+TCV	7	NONE	9	lung	GA	Lachmann et al. (1985)
BCG+TCV	148	NONE	145	colorectal	LS	Gray et al. (1989)
CPARV+TCV	46	NONE	49	lung	LS	Souter et al. (1981)
LEVA+CH	69	PBO+CH	71	ovarian	GA	Khoo et al. (1984)
LEVA+CH	15	CH	14	colorectal	GA	Sertoli et al. (1987)
LEVA(HD)+CH	132	CH	121	lung	LS	Davis et al. (1982)
LEVA(LD)+CH	61	CH	67	lung		
CPARV+LEVA	17	NONE+PBO	21	lung	LS	Fox et al. (1980)
BEST+CH	48	CH	53	acute nonlymphocytic leukaemia	LS	Ota et al. (1986)

Appendix 5.2: List of non-randomized cancer trials included in this survey

Test drug	Test patients evaluated	Control group	Control patients evaluated	Form of cancer	Outcome of scoring	Reference
aIFN	7	—	—	chronic myelogenous leukaemia	GA	Talpaz et al. (1983)
aIFN	30	—	—	hairy cell leukaemia	GA	Quesada et al. (1986a)
aIFN	14	—	—	ovarian	GA	Berek et al. (1985)
aIFN	19	—	—	cutaneous T-cell lymphoma	GA	Bunn et al. (1984)
aIFN	21	—	—	hairy cell leukaemia	HS	Jacobs et al. (1985)
aIFN	226	—	—	renal	LS	Umeda and Niijima (1986)
aIFN	22	—	—	pancreatic	LS	Eriksson et al. (1986)
aIFN	35	no IFN	30	osteosarcoma	LS	Strander et al. (1982)
aIFN	9	—	—	carcinoid	HS	Oberg et al. (1983)
aIFN	13	—	—	hairy cell leukaemia	GA	Thompson et al. (1985)
aIFN	7	—	—	hairy cell leukaemia	GA	Quesada et al. (1984)
aIFN	18	—	—	essential thrombocythaemia	GA	Giles et al. (1988)
aIFN	51	—	—	melanoma	GA	von Wussow et al. (1988)
aIFN	19	—	—	respiratory papilloma	GA	McCabe and Clark (1983)
aIFN	33	—	—	melanoma/colon #	HS	Kirkwood et al. (1985a)
aIFN	8	—	—	hairy cell leukaemia	HS	Ratain et al. (1985)
aIFN	26	—	—	Kaposi sarcoma	HS	de Wit et al. (1988)
aIFN	15	—	—	cervical	GA	Ikic et al. (1981)
aIFN	22	—	—	melanoma	GA	Dorval et al. (1986)
aIFN	38	—	—	breast/myeloma/lymphoma	LS	Gutterman et al. (1980)
aIFN	27	—	—	myeloma	HS	Quesada et al. (1986b)
aIFN	36	—	—	carcinoid	GA	Oberg et al. (1986)
aIFN	17	—	—	hairy cell leukaemia	LS	Worman et al. (1985)
aIFN	17	—	—	chronic myelogenous leukaemia	HS	Talpaz et al. (1986)
aIFN	37	—	—	non-Hodgkins lymphoma	HS	Foon et al. (1984)
aIFN	12	—	—	Kaposi sarcoma	GA	Krown et al. (1983)
aIFN+AZT	22	—	—	Kaposi sarcoma	HS	Kovacs et al. (1989)

Appendix 5.2: (cont)

Test drug	Test patients evaluated	Control group	Control patients evaluated	Form of cancer	Outcome of scoring	Reference
aIFN+DOX	15	—	—	renal	LS	Muss et al. (1985)
aIFN+ASP	29	—	—	renal	HS	Creagan et al. (1988)
bIFN	8	—	—	ovarian	LS	Rambaldi et al. (1985)
IL-2	7	—	—	melanoma/colorectal/ovarian	GA	Lotze et al. (1986)
IL-2+LAK	32	—	—	renal	HS	Fisher et al. (1988)
IL-2+LAK	23	—	—	glioma	LS	Yoshida et al. (1988)
IL-2+LAK/IL-2	152	—	—	colorectal/melanoma/lung renal/sarcoma/lymphoid	HS	Rosenberg et al. (1987)
IL-2+LAK	13	—	—	glioblastoma	GA	Merchant et al. (1988)
G-CSF	18	no G-CSF	17	urothelium (transitional cell)	LS	Gabrilove et al. (1988)
GM-CSF	19	no GM-CSF	23	breast/melanoma	GA	Brandt et al. (1988)
GM-CSF	14	no GM-CSF	86	various lymphoid	HS	Nemunaitis et al. (1988)
GM-CSF	14	no GM-CSF	12	sarcoma	GA	Antman et al. (1988)
TCV	78	—	—	breast	LS	Humphrey et al. (1984)
CH+BCG	62	—	—	acute leukaemia	LS	Bodey et al. (1981)
BCGex/Li/MNCT	11	—	—	hairy cell leukaemia	LS	Quesada et al. (1981)*
OK432	12	—	—	lung	LS	Uchida and Micksche (1983)
131-I Ab	79	—	—	hepatic	LS	Order et al. (1985)
131-I Ab	37	—	—	Hodgkins	LS	Lenhard et al. (1985)
anti-Id	10	—	—	B-cell malignancies	HS	Meeker et al. (1985)
TP-1	8	CH/none	24	melanoma	LS	Bernengo et al. (1983)

\# = Also one patient each with: renal/osteosarcoma/myeloma/Hodgkins/histiocytic lymphous/mycosis fungoides
* = Comparative trial of several test drugs; no control group used

Key to Appendices

aIFN	=	alpha-interferon (Leukocyte or recombinant sources)
anti-Id	=	anti-idiotypic antibodies
ASP	=	aspirin
AZT	=	azido-deoxythymidine
BCG	=	*Bacillus Calmette-Guerin*
BCGextr	=	extract or derivative of BCG e.g. Methanol extraction residue (MER) or cell wall skeleton (CWS)
BEST	=	Bestatin
bIFN	=	beta-interferon
CH	=	chemotherapy
CPARV	=	*Corynebacterium parvum*
DOX	=	Doxorubicin
gIFN	=	gamma-interferon
G-CSF	=	granulocyte colony stimulating factor
GM-CSF	=	granulocyte-macrophage colony stimulating factor
H	=	hormonal therapy (e.g. antioestrogens or androgens)
HD	=	high dose
IL-2	=	interleukin 2
LAK	=	lymphokine activated killer cells
LD	=	low dose
LEVA	=	Levamisole
Li	=	lithium
MELPH	=	Melphalan
MNCT	=	mononuclear cell transfer
NOC	=	*Nocardia rubra*
NOCextr	=	extract or derivative of *Nocardia rubra* e.g. cell wall skeleton (CWS)
NONE	=	control group received 'no treatment'
OK432	=	*Streptococcus pyogenes* A3
PBO	=	Placebo
PRED	=	Prednisone
PROPI	=	*Propionibacterium granulosum*
TCV	=	tumour cell vaccine
T'CYCLINE	=	tetracycline
TP-1	=	Thymostimulin
131-I Ab	=	antibodies conjugated with radioactive iodine
x + y	=	patients received both drugs x and y
x/y	=	two treatment groups: one received drug x, the other drug y
CH+/−H	=	two treatment groups: one received chemotherapy and hormonal therapy, the other chemotherapy alone
CH+/−H*	=	three treatment groups: two with different chemotherapy regimens and one with combined chemotherapy and hormonal therapy

6

Immunological prevention and treatment of infectious disease

Introduction

The range of infectious agents which afflicts mankind includes: bacteria, fungi, viruses, protozoa, and helminths. Great strides in the elimination of the infectious threat have been made in the developed world and, through the guidance of the World Health Organisation (WHO), are being applied to the less developed countries. Not all of these advances involve medical intervention. Probably the greatest advance in reducing the incidence of infection in London, for example, was the construction of the sewerage and fresh water systems in the 19th century. The supply of clean water remains a priority for the WHO in the developing countries. This is just one way in which the incidence of disease is being reduced by minimizing human exposure to infectious agents. Another is to interrupt the life-cycle of parasites by eradicating organisms which act as hosts.

The technique of vaccination, introduced by Jenner almost 200 years ago and greatly developed 100 years later by Pasteur in Paris and von Behring and Kitasato in Berlin, is responsible for reducing the incidence of infectious disease more than any other medical intervention as illustrated by, for example, the virtual disappearance of polio from the UK. The development and application of vaccines continues apace, recent successes including the hepatitis B vaccine (reviewed by Fagan and Eddleston 1985) and the WHO smallpox eradication programme.

Regarding the treatment of infection, the discovery of penicillin by Fleming and its clinical development by Florey and Chain were followed by the establishment of a vast antibiotics industry which has provided an invaluable armoury for combatting infection by bacteria and fungi. Latterly, Acyclovir has, at last, provided a direct anti-viral agent. However, the current threat from infectious disease should not be underestimated. The subtle implications of some chronic viral infections are only now being elucidated, whilst parasitic infection remains a major cause of morbidity in the less developed world. Bacterial resistance to antibiotics has been observed and septic shock remains a life-threatening complication of overwhelming bacterial infection. The AIDS virus provides the clearest example of man's impotence, albeit temporary, in the treatment of infection.

Chronic infection may be the result or the cause of immunodeficiency. In the latter case, the induction of immunodeficiency by the pathogen represents an evolutionary adaption to permit survival and reproduction in the host. A particularly successful form of chronic infection is that achieved by the protozoan and helminthic parasites. Ottesen and Sher (1988) reviewed the extraordinary range of means by which these organisms may outwit the immune system in order to survive. These include molecular mimicry of host antigens (schistosomes), acquisition of antigens from the host, the parasite demonstrably lacking the appropriate DNA blueprint (schistosomes), rapid turnover and variation of surface molecules (trypanosomes), proteolytic cleavage of IgG when it attaches to surface antigens (*Trypanosoma cruzi*), secretion of complement-depleting agents (*Taenia*), and evasion of the immune system by assuming an intracellular location (*Trypanosoma*, *Plasmodium*, *Leishmania*). Immune complexes are also observed (*Plasmodium*, *Trypanosoma*) with attendant disease (glomerulonephritis and vasculitis). In some cases, immune complexes could represent the attachment of shed antigen to antibodies, thus actively shielding the parasite from the humoral immune response. It is conceivable that useful lessons about the survival of tumours may be learnt from a study of parasites.

It may well be a drastic over-simplification, however, to regard the interaction between pathogen and the immune system as purely immunosuppressive. Ottesen and Sher point out that the life-cycle of the parasite requires that it survive for a long period of time within the host and therefore overwhelming, lethal, parasitic infection must be avoided. The immune response may be modulated so that parasites are destroyed whenever a threshold level of infection is exceeded.

The fascinating and important emerging field of viral immunopathology suggests that the interaction of virus and host immunity can be complex, particularly for those viruses which are capable of integration into host DNA. For example, some viruses may be aetiological agents in cancer or autoimmune disease as well as causing either acute self-limiting or chronic infectious disease. The ultimate outcome of infection may depend upon the nature of the immune response to which the virus is initially exposed and/or the presence of cofactors. This may be the case for Epstein–Barr virus (EBV). Initial infection in childhood may be asymptomatic or result in infectious mononucleosis (commonly called 'glandular fever'). Although symptoms may in due course

disappear, lifelong infection is established and EBV has been impli-
cated in the aetology of Burkitt's lymphoma and nasopharyngeal carcinoma (Thompson *et al*. 1988). An association of EBV with rheumatoid
arthritis is also under investigation (Lotz and Vaughan 1988). Burkitt's
lymphoma is especially common in Africa, whilst nasopharyngeal carcinoma is prevalent in Asia. By contrast, infectious mononucleosis is
observed throughout the world. This suggests that cofactors are involved in determining the long term outcome of EBV infection.

One possible explanation for the variable outcome of infection would
be the availability to the virus of several developmental pathways, each
subject to different forms of immune constraint, the virus progressing
along the line of least resistance. The existence of predisposing features, such as the observed correlation of susceptibility to some diseases with the presence of certain genetic markers associated with the
immune system (e.g. HLA), could reflect an involvement of these
markers (or the product of a linked gene) in determining the relative
resistance of each pathway. Cofactors could influence the outcome of
infection by modulating the relative immunological resistance of the
developmental pathways.

Immunological agents have been applied to infectious disease to
provide prophylaxis (active or passive immunization) or treatment. In
the latter case, immunological agents have been used not only in
diseases where there is a demonstrable immunodeficiency but also in
those lacking clear evidence of immunodeficiency in the hope that
boosting the immune system will accelerate recovery. For the purposes
of this survey, active immunization was considered separately (see
below) from passive immunization and treatment of ongoing disease
(p. 130) because of the special problems associated with vaccine trials,
especially those undertaken on large populations in remote locations.

Active immunization

Special features of vaccine trials

There are a number of special problems facing the clinical trialist
venturing into the evaluation of a new vaccine. These include:

1. The treatment groups should be comparable in terms of exposure
   to the pathogen of interest. This is not relevant to some studies
   such as the reactivation of latent CMV due to transplantation
   immunosuppression. It is relevant when, for example, infection
   requires an insect bite and some participants use insect repellents

whilst others do not. It will be necessary to demonstrate that the use of repellents occurred equally in the two treatment groups. If a trial is performed in two areas where the probability of exposure may be different, then it will be necessary to show that the participants from the various treatment groups were distributed equally between the two locations or that the level of exposure in the two areas was in fact the same. Otherwise, the outcome and the level of exposure (or the use of insect repellents) must both be included in some form of multivariate analysis (see question 27 of the scoring system).

2. The trials may be very large, involving many thousands of participants because of a low natural incidence of the disease in the general population. The alternative is to find a high-risk group. If a large trial is decided upon then it is especially vital that a simple and objective endpoint is clearly defined, because the participants will be assessed by numerous clinicians and hence there is considerable scope for variation in the results. This will effectively reduce statistical power by reducing the 'signal to noise ratio' of the data. If the endpoints are well defined and a minimum of subjective judgement is required, then the power of the trial will effectively be higher. Where endpoints cannot be completely objective, measures should be taken to enhance the standardization of data by, for example, having an independent monitoring committee which reviews each case and confirms the outcome according to a set of standard criteria. Alternatively, a conference of all participating clinicians could be held periodically to review the latest batch of diagnoses (see questions 2, 12, 22, and 26).

3. Some vaccine trials are conducted far from well equipped laboratories or sophisticated diagnostic equipment. The clinical endpoints therefore need to be based upon the use of simple techniques. Laboratory samples will need to be transported, sometimes over considerable distances in hot climates. It is essential that any effects of the transport system upon the reliability of the results is carefully checked (see questions 2, 22, 23, and QC(iv)).

4. The considerable expense of a large trial makes it especially important to ensure that the number of patients enrolled will provide a statistically sound result. It would be a great waste to vaccinate and monitor several thousand patients only to conclude that failure to observe a difference between treatment and control groups could

be due to type II error. Power calculations must be performed. It cannot simply be assumed that enrolling thousands of patients will give adequate statistical power because this depends upon the number of evaluable events as well as the number of patients. Sequential designs may have a role here in ensuring a statistically sound result with the minimum number of patients. Such methods involve the addition of each new outcome to an ongoing statistical analysis with an independent committee empowered to stop the trial according to pre-set rules such as the attainment of a particular level of significance. Such methods are necessarily complex, in order to guard against the problems associated with multiple looks at data, and must only be conducted by a qualified statistician. Attempts to attain a statistically sound result may be confounded if a large number of patients are lost to follow-up due to out-migration from the region. Locations should therefore be chosen with stable populations, according to recent demographic data (see questions 8, 10, 11, 30, and 32).

5. In order to generalize the results obtained, it is important to know how the selected population relates to the general population. For example, in some countries, those who have access to healthcare services, and are more likely to be enrolled, may represent a more affluent subgroup and the results would not necessarily generalize to a poorer, less well-fed population. Alternatively, an international agency may target their trial upon a less well-off group where the observed efficacy of the vaccine may be reduced due to malnutrition immunosuppression (see question 14).

6. Similarly it is important to be able to relate the dosage regimen received by the trial participants to the rigours of everyday usage. Whilst trial supplies may arrive via a strict 'cold chain', this may not be the case when the vaccine enters routine use. Repeat vaccinations may be missed or delayed. It would therefore be helpful if the trialists reported efficacy not just in those who received the entire regimen but also in those who received partial or interrupted regimens. Alternatively, trialists could give the percentages of patients who received 100, 90, or 80 per cent etc. of the regimen (see questions 17 and 19).

Outcome of scoring vaccine trials

Fifteen vaccine RCTs, involving 136,367 evaluable patients, were included in this survey. The scores achieved by the 15 RCTs ranged from

36 to 67 per cent, with a mean of 52 per cent and a median of 53 per cent. There was no correlation ($R^2 = 0.095$) between score and year of publication, which ranged from 1980 to 1988. Table 6.1 shows which questions most frequently achieved each possible score.

Vaccine NRCTs were not surveyed for two reasons. Firstly, NRCTs carried out early in the development of a vaccine usually concentrate upon immunogenicity, which is quickly and easily monitored, rather than clinical endpoints which often involve long-term follow-up of a large number of patients for a small number of events. Secondly, in situations where randomized trials are impracticable for a study of clinical efficacy, there is a well-established alternative in the form of case-control studies. The relative merits of RCTs and case-control studies have been reviewed by Smith (1988). Essentially, a case-control study involves enrolling patients who have contracted the disease in question and determining whether or not they have been vaccinated. Meanwhile, non-diseased persons, matched as closely as possible in terms of age, sex, and other confounding factors such as nutritional status and exposure to the pathogen, are also questioned to determine whether or not they were ever vaccinated. A 2×2 table is derived, of cases and controls versus vaccination or no vaccination, from which the protective efficacy of the vaccine can be calculated. Such methods avoid the problems inherent in other epidemiological methods such as time-course or retrospective cohort studies. The quality of case-control studies is dictated by a distinct set of sampling rules which are outside the scope of this book. Such studies were not therefore included in this survey.

Occasionally, however, a NRCT is the method of choice when randomization to a non-treatment control group is not ethical and consistency of the endpoint has been demonstrated throughout the population for many years. The latter point means that patients in the two treatment groups start from an equal baseline probability of trial failure regardless of how they are allocated to the two groups. This was the case for the incidence of the hepatitis B carrier state in Taiwanese infants (Beasley *et al.* 1983). In this trial of combined active and passive immunization, the treatment group was compared with a composite control group of historical cases and persons who refused participation in the active treatment arm of the trial. This study is discussed further on page 140.

Questions which usually scored '2'

Endpoints were generally clearly defined (question 2; points (2) and (3) on p. 117). For example, Szmuness *et al.* (1982) defined three

Table 6.1   Score frequencies for each question for the vaccine RCTs

Question number	Subject of question	Score frequency (per cent)			Sample[*] number
		2	1	0	
Questions which usually scored '2'					
2	Definition of endpoints	93.33	0.00	6.67	15
3	Informed consent before randomization	86.67	6.67	6.67	15
5	Blindness of patients to treatment	86.67	6.67	6.67	15
6	Blindness of clinicians to treatment	86.67	6.67	6.67	15
7	Blindness to ongoing results	53.33	0.00	46.67	15
12	Reporting of patient selection criteria	53.33	33.33	13.33	15
13	Reporting of patient numbers	53.33	46.67	0.00	15
15	Patient withdrawal log	75.00	0.00	25.00	8
17	Reporting of dosage regimen	86.67	13.33	0.00	15
18	Identity of comparator in blind studies	50.00	7.14	42.86	14
19	Interruptions to drug administration	41.67	25.00	33.33	12
22	Objectivity of clinical monitoring	86.67	13.33	0.00	15
27	Baseline comparison of patients	66.67	20.00	13.33	15
28	Reporting of results	80.00	13.33	6.67	15
Questions which usually scored '1'					
8	Choice of statistical methods	13.33	46.67	40.00	15
16	Exclusion of concomitant diseases	0.00	53.33	46.67	15
23	Relevance of immunological monitoring	0.00	100.00	0.00	13
24	Close monitoring for adverse events	6.67	80.00	13.33	15
29	Adverse event reporting	20.00	46.67	33.33	15
31	Statistical reporting	0.00	53.33	46.67	15
Questions which usually scored '0'					
1	Number of endpoints	13.33	40.00	46.67	15
4	Method of randomization	6.67	0.00	93.33	15
9	Homogeneity check on multicentre data	14.29	0.00	85.71	7
10	Trial size by power calculation	20.00	6.67	73.33	15
11	Other reason for trial size	25.00	8.33	66.67	12
14	Patient reject log	33.33	6.67	60.00	15
20	Exclusion of concomitant therapies	6.67	0.00	93.33	15
25	Adverse immunological event reporting	33.33	6.67	60.00	15
26	Uniformity of multicentre evaluations	14.29	0.00	85.71	7
30	Dropout accounting	21.43	35.71	42.86	14
32	Results in terms of trial size	0.00	7.14	92.86	14
Questions which were 'NA' in every case					
21	length of washout in crossover studies				

[*]Sample number = the number of trials scored minus the number for which the question was not applicable

types of event related to hepatitis B virus (HBV) infection. These were: 'hepatitis B', 'HBV infection with minimal liver damage' and 'anti-HBc seroconversion only'. Each was defined in terms of a threshold number of consecutive blood samples in which specified antigens or antibodies or enzyme activities were observed. For example, a patient was considered to have hepatitis B if two or more consecutive blood samples were positive for HBsAg, or anti-HBc, or both *and* two or more consecutive blood samples had alanine aminotransferase values above the upper limit of normal ($\geq$ 45 IU per litre) *and* one or more of the blood samples had alanine aminotransferase values at least twice the upper limit of normal ($\geq$ 90 IU per litre). The time interval between blood samples was specified as monthly unless an HBV event was detected, in which case samples were taken every 2 weeks until the event had been characterized. The trialists go on to say that all such data were reviewed by an independent panel of experts and a consensus reached on all cases included in the analysis (see point 2 on p. 117). Definitions were also given of 'good' and 'fair' anti-HBs responses to the vaccine. Similar endpoints were used by, for example, Francis *et al.* (1982) and Szmuness *et al.* (1980) and require ready access to high-capacity laboratory facilities. Simpler endpoints, more suited to trials conducted away from such facilities, usually comprise a set of simple clinical criteria, requiring the minimum of equipment, backed up by laboratory tests on a small number of samples taken only from those who met the clinical criteria. For example, in the Gambian Rotavirus study (Hanlon *et al.* 1987), diarrhoea was defined as: 'the passage of three or more loose stools in any 24 hour period . . . classed as severe if its duration was greater than 24 hours and it was associated with one or more of the following: passage of six or more stools in 24 hours, vomiting, rectal temperature over 38 °C, clinical dehydration'. Stools from such patients were examined at the MRC laboratories in The Gambia to determine the presence or absence of rotavirus. Similarly, in the US Army study of Japanese encephalitis in Thailand (Hoke *et al.* 1988), cases of febrile central nervous system disease were sought (temperature >38 °C, lethargy, obtundation or coma) and samples of blood and cerebrospinal fluid (CSF) were taken for determination of antibody levels (blood and CSF) and leucocyte counts (CSF).

The heavy reliance upon antigen titres and enzyme activities amongst the studies surveyed ensured that question 22 (points 2 and 3 on p. 117), relating to the objectivity of monitoring, usually scored '2'. Other firm endpoints included death (Clemens *et al.* 1988) and histological studies of skin lesion biopsy specimens (Antunes *et al.* 1986). Whilst some studies relied upon participants who developed relevant symptoms presenting themselves to a clinic, others employed field workers who visited the trial participants in their homes. For example, in the Venezuelan rotavirus study (Flores *et al.* 1987) 247 infants were visited daily in the first week after vaccination and twice weekly thereafter. Some monitoring efforts can only be described as heroic, such as the weekly or biweekly home visits to the 200 000 inhabitants of the Matlab delta in Bangladesh (Clemens *et al.* 1988)! In the US Army study of Japanese encephalitis in Thailand (Hoke *et al.* 1988), a description of the disease was broadcast daily throughout the province to call forth suspected cases. At the end of each epidemic period, a census of every participant was carried out to ensure that no cases had been missed.

The majority of the 15 studies surveyed were performed double-blind against placebo (questions 3, 5, and 6). One trial (Hanlon *et al.* 1987) was a special case, having two treatment groups each with oral treatments administered blind, and a third group which included an intramuscular treatment and could not therefore be administered blind. Significantly, many trialists reported the identity of the placebo and active treatments (e.g. Coutinho *et al.* 1983 and Wong *et al.* 1984), whilst others reported generating a placebo by running the vaccine production procedure without the pathogen from which the vaccine would normally be produced. For example, Vesikari *et al.* (1984) produced a bovine rotavirus vaccine in primary monkey kidney cells, the placebo being made using uninfected primary monkey kidney cells. One trial of killed whole cell cholera vaccine used *E. coli* K12 as a placebo (Clemens *et al.* 1988). Thus question 18, relating to identity of the placebo, scored '2' most frequently. The majority of trialists reported that they had not had access to the ongoing results of the study and that the code had been broken only at the end of the trial (question 7).

The combination of the above trial features: clear endpoint definitions, objective monitoring and blindness go a long way towards ensuring that the results from these studies can be relied upon. As was observed for the cancer studies, the questions dealing with such basic trial features as patient selection (question 12; point 2 on p. 117), the number of patients enrolled and evaluated (question 13), the dosage regimen (question 17), and the reporting of results (question 28) usually scored '2'. Trials of hepatitis vaccine selected high-risk participants including children of hepatitis carriers (Wong *et al.* 1984), haemodialysis staff (Szmuness *et al.* 1982), or homosexuals (Coutinho *et al.* 1983).

The majority of studies reported relevant baseline information about their patient populations (question 27). As discussed above (point 1 on p. 116), in a prophylactic study it is important to demonstrate that the study groups were exposed equally to the pathogen. The simplest way to achieve this is to enrol the population of a single geographical region where a predictable annual epidemic occurs (e.g. the Gambian rotavirus study (Hanlon *et al.* 1987)). In a trial of hepatitis vaccine amongst American homosexuals (Szmuness *et al.* 1980), the mean number of sexual partners during the previous 6 months was shown to be the same for the participants in the two treatment groups, thus suggesting the risk of encountering hepatitis-bearing partners was the same for both groups. In the Brazilian Army trial of a leishmania vaccine (Antunes *et al.* 1986), detailed data about the time spent in the jungle and the locations visited by each military unit were obtained from the Army Central Office in Manaus.

Amongst the 15 studies surveyed, 8 reported patients being withdrawn from the analysis. The reasons for withdrawal were usually given (question 15). For example, Hanlon *et al.* (1987) reported that 80 vaccinees were excluded from efficacy analysis because they were absent from the area during the annual epidemic which was the *raison d'etre* of the trial. They were, however, included in the analysis of serological data. Szmuness *et al.* (1982) reported that two vaccinees had transient anti-HBc events which were not regarded as bona fide hepatitis events and were excluded from the analysis. The trialists point out that this did not bias the trial in favour of the vaccine because both occurred in the control group. Drop-out accounting was generally much less well done and most frequently scored '0' (see below).

Twelve of the fifteen vaccine trials involved the administration of more than one injection. Most of these reports included information about interruptions in the regimen and/or whether or not participants who received only part of the planned regimen were included in the analysis (question 19; point 6 on p. 118). For example, the analyses of the Bangladeshi Cholera trial (Clemens *et al.* 1988) and the French hepatitis trial (Crosnier *et al.* 1981) included only those who had received all three doses of the planned regimen, whilst the analysis of the Gambian rotavirus trial (Hanlon *et al.* 1987) included children who had received at least one of the three planned doses. Several trials clearly tabulated or listed the number of patients receiving each dose as well as the length of time between successive vaccinations as compared to the planned intervals in the protocol (e.g. Coutinho *et al.* 1983). This question usually scored '2'. Three studies involving only single doses were scored as 'not applicable'.

Questions which usually scored '1'

Regarding immunological monitoring (question 23; point 3 on p. 117),

13 trials reported the levels of specific antibody, this data often being used as a clinical diagnostic such as in the endpoint definitions for hepatitis studies. Some studies sought specific antibodies in locations other than serum which were relevant to the action of the vaccine. For example in the study of Japanese encephalitis (Hoke *et al.* 1988), specific antibodies were sought in the cerebrospinal fluid of suspected cases. The immune response to an infectious agent is multi-faceted, often involving more than the generation of antibodies. The reporting of specific antibodies alone was therefore assigned the score '1', although it is appreciated that large studies of clinical efficacy, some of which are conducted far from a laboratory, are not the place for in-depth immunological monitoring which can more satisfactorily be conducted on the smaller initial studies of immunogenicity and safety.

Four questions (16, 24, 25, and 29) deal with the detection and reporting of adverse events, of which all but question 25 scored '1'. Several studies, such as Vesikari *et al.* (1984) and Vesikari *et al.* (1985), excluded persons with chronic diseases from trial participation (question 16), whilst in other studies the general state of health of the participants could be inferred to some extent from the fact that they were working hospital staff (Szmuness *et al.* 1982) or undergoing military training, albeit as conscripts (Antunes *et al.* 1986). For question 24, several studies reported subjective events such as soreness or headache, although few reported laboratory monitoring of blood counts, renal function markers, etc. This is understandable in terms of the sheer scale and logistic problems of some vaccine studies, in-depth safety monitoring presumably having been undertaken in smaller studies earlier in the development of the vaccine. On the other hand, the large clinical efficacy studies provide an opportunity to pick up the low frequency adverse events that might be missed in the smaller studies. Laboratory monitoring should therefore be undertaken whenever trials are conducted in locations where the facilities are readily available. The reporting of adverse events (question 29) was often rather sparse and lacking in detail in terms of duration and severity of the event. Wong *et al.* (1984) gave a fairly detailed account of their experience with a hepatitis vaccine, reporting that 'the babies were healthy and had only the usual intercurrent illnesses. At all times the weight and height percentiles of the babies were within normal limits for their age and sex . . . No serious side-effects from the injections were noticed.' The trialists go on to mention the side-effects they did observe, such as fever and swelling at the site of injection, together with an indication of the severity and duration of each. Hanlon *et al.* (1987) stated simply and definitively that 'no vaccine side-effects were observed' with their rotavirus vaccine.

As explained in Chapter 4, the statement about statistical methods in the 'Methods' section of the paper should include a brief sentence indicating how the chosen method copes with any peculiarities of the data or the study design (question 8). The commonest fault was the use of the *t*-test without any indication of whether or not the distribution of the data was suited to such a method. Some studies had more than two treatment groups but gave no indication of how the chosen methods of analysis would cope with this design feature. For example, to state that the Chi-square test is to be used when there are three treatment groups (A, B, C) and two outcomes begs the question of whether a 3×2 comparison (A vs B vs C) *or* three 2×2 comparisons (A vs B; B vs C; A vs C) *or* pooled data comparisons (A + B vs C *or* B + C vs A *or* A + C vs B) are envisaged. If, subsequently, the result of just one comparison is reported then the reader is left unclear as to how this selection of possible comparisons was arrived at. This situation occurred in Hanlon *et al.* (1987), where the A + C vs B comparison was reported as having 'just reached statistical significance ($p<0.05$)'. Some studies stated in the 'Methods' section how they coped with several treatment groups. For example, in Clemens *et al.* (1988), the trialists stated that 'two-group contrasts . . . were statistically appraised only if the overall three group comparison was significant at $p <0.05$'.

Some prophylactic studies benefit from being analysed in terms of a Kaplan–Meier plot and logrank (or similar) test which displays the timecourse of events and accounts for dropouts. For example in Szmuness *et al.* (1982), a life-table plot of the incidence of HBV events showed that whereas the placebo group events were fairly evenly distributed throughout the 2-year follow-up period, the small number of vaccine group events nearly all took place in the first few months. In some studies (e.g. Hanlon *et al.* 1987), however, the time course is not of interest, efficacy being determined by the overall incidence of disease during a brief epidemic period (3 months in this case) and in such studies a simple Chi-square test suffices unless there are other reasons for more complex statistics.

The reporting of statistical analyses (question 31) scored '1' most frequently due to several studies including confidence intervals, usually in association with estimates of protective efficacy. In Clemens *et al.* (1988), for example, the protective efficacy of the killed whole cell cholera vaccine with B-subunit was quoted as 26 per cent with confidence limits of 12–38 per cent. Many papers, however, quoted the attainment of *p*-value thresholds (usually $p <0.05$) rather than the actual values. In one study, with three treatment groups, it was stated that the incidence of a side-effect in one treatment group was 'not significant' compared to the control group, whilst comparison of the second treatment group with the control group yielded '$p < 0.05$'. Clearly, this could be a dangerous statement if the p-value for the first comparison was 0.055 and for the second it was 0.045. The value $p = 0.05$ is wrongly regarded as some kind of magical threshold whereby results have quite different properties on either side of this figure. On the contrary, the p-value represents the probability of the observed difference being due to chance. It follows that both comparisons, if they did indeed have the values suggested, would be worrying. Fortunately in this case (Hoke *et al.* 1988) the trialists also included the sample numbers and the percentage incidence of side-effects for all three groups, so readers could calculate the precise p-values if they wished. However, such information is not always supplied in published reports.

Questions which usually scored '0'

Many of the vaccine trials surveyed had several endpoints (question 1). This is perhaps understandable in terms of the size, cost, and logistic complexity of some vaccine trials, it being desirable to gain as much information as possible from the population being studied. Equally, it is a shame if any shadow of statistical doubt can be cast upon the results obtained from such trials. It would therefore be desirable for trialists to indicate at the outset which endpoint is to be considered as the primary one, the others providing suggestive or supportive, but not pivotal, data. Alternatively, the kind of statistical methods referred to by Pocock (1987) for coping with multiple endpoints could be used.

Only one trial (Antunes *et al.* 1986) gave an account of the randomization procedure used in the trial (question 4) and of the measures to ensure the blindness of treatment allocation. In order to make it especially difficult for treatment allocation to be guessed, drug vials were provided labelled in eight different ways, four of which corresponded to active treatment and four to placebo. Randomization and the labelling of vials was carried out by a person who had no contact with those responsible for evaluating patients.

Of the seven multicentre studies surveyed, only one (Francis *et al.* 1982) presented the results by centre, thus showing that the overall outcome was not due to one aberrant centre (question 9). In this example, the incidence of hepatitis at all five centres was above 0.09 for placebo patients and below 0.085 for vaccine recipients. This study also reported that all samples for serological testing and liver enzyme determinations were shipped to a central laboratory, thus ensuring standardization of results (question 26; point 2 on p. 117).

As discussed in Chapter 4, a clinical trial is a statistical sampling exercise and it is essential that the size of the trial be determined at the outset, preferably by means of a statistical power calculation. Questions 10 and 11 address this issue, whilst question 32 relates to whether the concept of sample size was considered *post-hoc*, in the discussion section, when no reason had been given at the outset or whenever actual and projected results differed markedly (see point 4 on p. 117). Of the 15 vaccine RCTs considered here, 4 included a power calculation at the outset, 4 gave other reasons for trial size and 7 gave no reason whatsoever. For example, Crosnier *et al.* (1981) stated that '... a minimum of 61 participants per group would be necessary to demonstrate a reduction of the incidence rate of HBV infection from 15 per cent to 1 per cent during a period of 12 months with type I error alpha = 5 per cent and type II error beta = 5 per cent'. (In this case the actual results were so close to the projected ones, 12.3 and 3.6 per cent, respectively, that question 32 was regarded as not applicable.) For three studies (Clemens *et al.* 1988, Hoke *et al.* 1988, and Hanlon *et al.* 1987), trial size was dictated by the population of a geographical region. One report (Antunes *et al.* 1986), concerned vaccination of Brazilian army conscripts against cutaneous leishmaniasis, and the trialists mentioned a much reduced incidence of disease in the control group as possibly being responsible for failure to observe efficacy in two or three conscript subgroups.

Of the three studies involving entire populations, two were enormous with over 60 000 participants each. Such large trials are not, however, automatically assured of high statistical power if the number of evaluable events is very low. For example, the US Army trial of Japanese encephalitis virus vaccine in Thailand (Hoke *et al.* 1988) enrolled 22 080 persons on the bivalent vaccine, 21 628 persons on the monovalent vaccine and 21 516 persons on placebo. The number of cases of Japanese encephalitis observed in each group was: 11 on placebo and 1 each for the two vaccine groups! The proportion of placebo recipients not getting Japanese encephalitis was therefore 99.95 per cent and the proportion of vaccinated patients remaining disease free was 99.995 per cent. If a trial were to be designed on the basis of these figures then a power calculation of the form described in Chapter 4 indicates that such a trial would have just slightly better than 80 per cent statistical power for detecting this difference as significant at the 5 per cent level despite the vast patient numbers.

The use of an external committee to decide when a trial should stop (see point 4 on p. 117) was employed by an American study of hepatitis vaccine on homosexuals (Francis *et al.* 1982). This trial did not employ a sequential method of analysis (i.e. each new event added to an ongoing analysis) but rather, the committee re-analysed the data at three time points during the trial. On this basis a stricter level of significance than $p = 0.05$ should be sought and the criteria for stopping the trial should be decided at the outset. Although the stopping rules were not given in the paper, it is apparent that a high level of significance was sought, the overall result (58 events amongst 714 vaccinees and 110 events amongst 688 placebo recipients) having a p-value of <0.00001 by the Mantel–Cox method.

Six studies included a reject log (question 14; point 5 on p. 118), thus giving some indication of how the selected population related to the general population. For example in a trial of hepatitis vaccine (Wong *et al.* 1984) in which 189 of 216 available babies were entered, the reasons for non-enrolment included: eight with birthweight less than 2500 g, eight with Apgar score less than 7, two with congenital abnormalities, one stillborn, one born after prolonged rupture of membranes, one brought to the hospital 3 hours after birth, and six withdrawn by their parents before treatment commenced. Studies which set out to enrol the entire population of a region do not always succeed in doing so, in which case a reject log should be included. In the Bangladeshi cholera vaccine study (Clemens *et al.* 1988) the trialists were unable to enrol 31 238 persons (25 per cent of the available population) because they were absent or refused to participate, whilst a further 3201 persons (2.6 per cent of the available population) were either pregnant or too ill to leave their beds. Several reports included background information on the geography and socio-economic status of the region as well as the general epidemiology of the disease under study. Such information is valuable in setting the trial in context and facilitating generalization of the results.

The possible interference of prior or concomitant immunosuppressive medications (question 20) was considered by the trialists in the Brazilian Army leishmaniasis study (Antunes *et al.* 1986) in terms of antigenic competition by recent prior vaccines to yellow fever, tetanus, and typhoid. Another possible concomitant drug problem would be the use of immunosuppressive drugs, such as Cyclosporin, by vaccine recipients in, for example, some of the studies of healthcare workers. Cyclosporin is being applied to an ever wider range of autoimmune and chronic inflammatory disorders (see Chapter 7) and there may not always be an obvious reason for suspecting that an apparently healthy individual was receiving immunosuppressive drugs. In the study of CMV vaccine in renal transplant patients (Plotkin *et al.* 1984), the vaccine was administered 8 weeks before the transplant, thus allowing time for antibody development before the use of immunosuppressive agents.

The possibility of adverse immunological events (question 25) was mentioned in only two trial reports. The possibility of anaphylactic reaction to Japanese encephalitis virus vaccine was discussed by Hoke *et al.* (1988) and was actively investigated. No cases were detected. Reference was made in Maupas *et al.* (1981) to previous work indicating no evidence of autoimmunity arising from the use of hepatitis vaccine. This paper also refers to there being 'no local or general reactions' to the vaccine. Statements such as 'no vaccine side-effects were observed' (Hanlon *et al.* 1987) or 'the babies were healthy and had only the usual intercurrent illnesses' (Wong *et al.* 1984) can presumably be taken to mean that no adverse immunological events were seen. The possibility of adverse immunological events was rarely specifically considered, however, and the usual score for this question was '0'.

As explained in Chapter 4, it is important for the reader to have access to information about the number of patients who were censored due to unelapsed time or lost to follow-up (question 30; point 4 on p. 117) for reasons such as lack of efficacy, side-effects, or unacceptability of the dosage regimen. Szmuness *et al.* (1982) provides a good example of drop-out accounting. In this study of hepatitis vaccination of dialysis unit staff, 383 of 865 participants (44 per cent) were lost to follow-up over a two-year period. The numbers of drop-outs per treatment group were given (203 vaccine and 180 placebo) and reference was made to a life-table analysis which showed that the rate of drop-out in the treatment groups was not significantly different (a *p*-value and the name of the statistical test used should have been given here). The same baseline characteristics that were compared for the initial treatment groups were also compared for the drop-out populations for each group. The data were tabulated and it is apparent that the drop-out populations in each treatment group were similar to each other and, indeed, similar to the initial complete groups. The reason given for loss to follow-up of these participants was that most changed their jobs, and whilst it might have been useful to list the other reasons, or at least to state that no-one departed for medical reasons, it is clear from the whole picture that, as the trialists state: 'it is therefore unlikely that the loss of these subjects introduced any bias into the study results'. A Kaplan–Meier plot was used in this study to present the trial results over a two-year period and the number of participants per group at ten timepoints were indicated in a table across the top of the graph. Of 442 vaccine and 423 placebo participants at $t = 0$, 203 and 180 were lost to follow-up, respectively, as noted above. However, the number of participants at $t = 2$ years was 123 on vaccine and 135 on placebo. It follows that 116 vaccine and 108 placebo participants must have been

enrolled less than two years before the trial was written up and are thus
censored from the graphs due to unelapsed time. The trialists state that
participants were enrolled between September 1979 and March 1981.
The date of publication is December 1982, which is indeed less than
two years after enrolment ceased. Drop-out accounting was not usually
carried out clearly, however, and the most usual score for this question
was '0'. Regarding choice of geographical location on the basis of
population stability, the location of the Senegalese hepatitis study
(Maupas *et al.* 1981) was selected on this basis.

QC questions
None of the 15 reports of vaccine RCTs mentioned data auditing or
questioning of the clinicians or participants in blind studies as to which
treatment group they thought particular participants were in. QC
checks for any effects of sample transportation upon the reliability of
the laboratory results were not mentioned.

Passive immunization and drug therapy

Forty clinical trials, comprising 23 RCTs (involving 1639 evaluable
patients) and 17 NRCTs (involving 642 evaluable patients) were included in this survey.

Outcome of scoring

RCTs
The scores achieved by the RCTs ranged from 18.5 to 68 per cent, with
a mean of 44.9 per cent and a median of 43 per cent. There was no
correlation ($R^2 = 0.078$) between score and year of publication, which
ranged from 1980 to 1989. Table 6.2 shows which questions most
frequently achieved each possible score. Two of the RCTs were performed on AIDS patients and these are also considered on p. 140.

Questions which usually scored '2'   For most of the trials included in this
survey, it was quite clear what was being monitored and, where necessary, endpoints were usually defined (question 2). In a study of pooled
CMV-immune serum, for example, Winston *et al.* (1982) diagnosed
CMV infection if CMV was isolated from cultures (of throat washings,
urine, buffy coat, biopsy, or autopsy material) or there was a fourfold
increase in CMV complement fixation antibody titre or both. The CMV
infection was considered symptomatic if the culture or serological result

Table 6.2 Score frequencies for each question for the infection RCTs

Question number	Subject of question	Score frequency (per cent)			Sample* number
		2	1	0	
Questions which usually scored '2'					
2	Definition of endpoints	65.22	17.39	17.39	23
3	Informed consent before randomization	69.57	0.00	30.43	23
5	Blindness of patients to treatment	69.57	0.00	30.43	23
6	Blindness of clinicians to treatment	69.57	8.70	21.74	23
12	Reporting of patient selection criteria	52.17	47.83	0.00	23
13	Reporting of patient numbers	78.26	17.39	4.35	23
15	Patient withdrawal log	35.71	28.57	35.71	14
17	Reporting of dosage regimen	82.61	13.04	4.35	23
22	Objectivity of clinical monitoring	73.91	21.74	4.35	23
23	Relevance of immunological monitoring	50.00	35.71	14.29	14
27	Baseline comparison of patients	78.26	13.04	8.70	23
28	Reporting of results	56.52	39.13	4.35	23
Questions which usually scored '1'					
8	Choice of statistical methods	5.26	47.37	47.37	19
24	Close monitoring for adverse events	21.74	52.17	26.09	23
29	Adverse event reporting	39.13	43.48	17.39	23
Questions which usually scored '0'					
1	Number of endpoints	8.70	8.70	82.61	23
4	Method of randomization	0.00	26.09	73.91	23
7	Blindness to ongoing results	21.74	0.00	78.26	23
9	Homogeneity check on multicentre data	0.00	0.00	100.00	9
10	Trial size by power calculation	0.00	0.00	100.00	23
11	Other reason for trial size	4.35	0.00	95.65	23
14	Patient reject log	8.70	0.00	91.30	23
16	Exclusion of concomitant diseases	17.39	4.35	78.26	23
18	Identity of comparator in blind studies	26.67	26.67	46.67	15
19	Interruptions to drug administration	9.09	9.09	81.82	22
20	Exclusion of concomitant therapies	17.39	34.78	47.83	23
21	Length of washout in crossover studies	0.00	0.00	100.00	1
25	Adverse immunological event reporting	26.09	30.43	43.48	23
26	Uniformity of multicentre evaluations	40.00	0.00	60.00	5
30	Dropout accounting	31.25	18.75	50.00	16
31	Statistical reporting	5.26	42.11	52.63	19
32	Results in terms of trial size	0.00	4.35	95.65	23

*Sample number = the number of trials scored minus the number for which the question was not applicable

was accompanied by pneumonia or a febrile illness that could not be explained by other causes. Interstitial pneumonia was indicated by tachypnea, hypoxaemia, fever, and interstitial pulmonary infiltrates shown on chest X-ray. The issue of defining whether death is related or unrelated to the disease of interest is discussed below in the context of sepsis.

Most of the trials were conducted double-blind (questions 3, 5, and 6). Amongst the open trials, the opportunity for bias was reduced in some by blind assessment of some of the endpoints, for example, Perrillo *et al.* (1988) (liver biopsy) and Silvestris *et al.* (1989) (T-cell numbers). Unfortunately, the related issues of randomization method (question 4), code-breaking (question 7) and identity of comparator (question 18) usually scored '0' and are discussed on p. 134. Nor in any of the open studies was it stated that informed consent was obtained without knowledge of randomization allocation (question 3), thus giving an opportunity for bias in these trials.

As was generally observed for the other therapeutic areas, questions dealing with basic issues such as patient selection criteria (question 12), the number of patients enrolled and evaluated (question 13), the dosage regimen (question 17), objectivity of clinical monitoring (question 22) and the reporting of results (question 28) usually scored well. Amongst the more difficult patient groups to define are those with sepsis, particularly in the neonate, and hence selection criteria should be especially clearly set out to enable meaningful comparisons to be made with other trials. Ziegler *et al.* (1982) selected adults or children who were severely ill, with recent deterioration (sudden high fever or hypothermia, hypotension or unexplained respiratory distress), and either good clinical evidence of an infection usually caused by gram-negative bacteria or an underlying disease predisposing to gram-negative infection. Haque and Zaidi (1988), in a study on neonates, defined sepsis thus: 'the presence of one or more clinical features such as lethargy, instability of temperature, glucose intolerance, increased gastric aspirate, hepatosplenomegaly, as well as any two of the following laboratory variables: immature-to-normal neutrophil ratio greater than 0.2, total white blood cell count less than 5.0 or greater than 30.0 $\times 10^9/l$ (uncorrected for age), platelet count less than 50.0 $\times 10^9/l$, and a positive blood or cerebrospinal fluid (CSF) culture'. When only clinical or biochemical criteria were met, 'suspected sepsis' was diagnosed. When cultures were also positive, 'proved sepsis' was diagnosed. Mean age at diagnosis in this study was 54.6 hours. Mortality provided an objective endpoint in both trials, and Ziegler *et al.* (1982) specified criteria for regarding the death as being related or unrelated to sepsis. Bacteraemic deaths were taken to be not only cases of irreversible bacteraemic shock but also deaths from non-infectious events that had occurred as a direct result of bacteraemia (e.g. myocardial infarction due to hypotension, or gastrointestinal, or cerebral haemorrhage due to disseminated intravascular coagulation). Deaths were not considered a direct result of bacteraemia if they took place several weeks after shock and infection had resolved (e.g. renal failure secondary to bacteraemic shock or continued dependence on respiratory assistance in patients with chronic lung disease who required tracheal intubation during an acute episode of bacteraemia).

The efficiency with which the reasons for patient withdrawal were reported (question 15) was very variable with almost equal numbers of studies scoring '2', '1', or '0'. It was often even less clear at what stage in the trial they were lost to follow-up or how the censored data was dealt with in the analysis (question 30).

Of the 11 trials in which immunological variables were monitored (question 23), most observed variables which were specifically relevant to the disease. For example, in a trial of Isoprinosine for herpes simplex infection, Kalimo *et al.* (1983) monitored lymphocyte transformation and antibody production in response to specific viral antigens. In a trial of transfer factor for the prevention of varicella zoster (VZV) in childhood leukaemia, Steele *et al.* (1980) employed skin testing with VZV antigen and monitored serum VZV antibodies.

The aim of eight of the studies was prophylaxis rather than treatment of ongoing infection. As discussed for vaccines, the level of exposure to the infectious agent must be shown to be equable for the treatment groups as part of the baseline comparison (question 27). This can be assumed for four of the prophylactic trials on reactivation of CMV in transplant recipients and a fifth involving experimental infection at the Common Cold Unit. Ausobsky *et al.* (1982) studied the incidence of post-operative infection in patients undergoing major laparotomies. In this single-centre trial all 166 patients were under the care of the same surgeon, thus giving an equal risk of infection for all patients. In a study of transfer factor for the prevention of chicken pox in leukaemic children, Steele *et al.* (1980) defined exposure predisposing to development of the disease as contact with siblings who had active lesions or playmates who were with patients indoors for more than 2 hours. Only cases meeting this criteria were evaluated. Farr *et al.* (1984) studied the ability of interferon to prevent colds acquired through natural exposure. Three hundred and four employees of a single company 'randomly distributed' through the workplace were studied.

Questions which usually scored '1'   Close monitoring for, and reporting
of, adverse events was frequently only partially accomplished in terms
of both questioning and laboratory monitoring of patients (question 24)
or the reporting of both severity and duration as well as incidence
(question 29). Questions 16 and 25 dealing with other aspects of adverse
event detection and monitoring usually scored '0' and are discussed
below. The appropriateness of statistical methods (question 8) scored '1'
and '0' with equal frequency according to the criteria set out in Chapter 4.

Questions which usually scored '0'   Most of the studies surveyed had
numerous endpoints and did not indicate which should be regarded as
the primary result. Exceptions included two studies with single endpoints: Steele *et al.* (1980) (incidence of chickenpox) and Haque and
Zaidi (1988) (death from sepsis).

None of the reports gave an account of the method of randomization
(question 4), although several made passing reference to random number tables or computer generated schemes. Perrillo *et al.* (1988) mentioned that the randomization scheme was kept by a research pharma-
cist who was unaware of clinical data on the patients. Scott *et al.* (1982)
paired patients according to age, sex, and pretrial neutralizing antibody
titre and then allocated them at random to active or control treatments.

Several trials reported that the code was broken only at the end of
the trial (question 7). In a multicentre trial, Ziegler *et al.* (1982) prepared data abstracts on each patient and these were discussed by a
committee, a consensus being reached prior to analysis. The trialists
state that all abstracts were completed and discussed before the code
was broken, and that no changes were made to the abstracts once
translation of the code had begun.

Of the 16 double-blind studies, four stated that the placebo was
identical in appearance to the active preparation (question 18). These
included three interferon trials, in which a human serum albumin
preparation was used, (Arvin *et al.* 1982; Farr *et al.* 1984; Scott *et al.*
1982) and the trial of Levamisole for prevention of post-operative infection (Ausobsky *et al.* 1982). The latter was administered by the oral
route, and perhaps in such cases it should be checked whether the
active and control preparations have similar flavours lest patients talk-
ing amongst themselves discern that some of them are getting, for
example, bitter pills and the others are getting sweet pills. If this were
to happen and then one of the 'bitter pill' recipients were to become
infected, there could be an effect upon the outcome of the other
patients, with the 'bitter pill' recipients convinced they are on placebo
and the 'sweet pill' recipients convinced they are on the active prepara-

tion. A placebo preparation coloured with a trace amount of riboflavin was used in a trial of transfer factor (Steele *et al.* 1980), although the authors do not state that the resulting preparation was identical. Pooled non-immune serum and immune serum obtained sequentially from the same donors (Ziegler *et al.* 1982) were assumed to be identical and no statement from the trialists was required (= 'NA').

None of the multicentre trials reported a homogeneity check on multicentre data (question 9), whilst only one reported on the stand-ardization of evaluations at the different centres (question 26). As discussed above, Ziegler *et al.* (1982) prepared data abstracts on each patient in a multicentre trial which were discussed by a committee and a consensus reached prior to code-breaking and analysis. [Several multi-centre trials with very routine endpoints were not regarded as requiring standardization (= 'NA')].

None of the 23 RCTs surveyed used a power calculation to determine trial size (question 10) and only one (Reilly *et al.* 1986) gave another reason for trial size (question 11). This was a trial of beta-interferon in epidemic adenovirus conjunctivitis and the size of the trial was there-fore determined by the number of patients who presented during the epidemic. The trialists took active steps to discourage attendance at the eye hospital because of the suspected nosocomial origin of the epidemic. This resulted in the trialists concluding that the study was too small to make any statistically valid conclusion about the efficacy of beta-interferon in this condition (question 32).

Of the 19 'high-score' or 'grey-area' RCTs, 5 showed no difference between active and control treatments, in terms of efficacy. In an attempt to probe the scope for type II statistical error (the probability of concluding that two treatments have the same efficacy when there is really a difference), power calculations were performed according to the method described in Chapter 4. The outcome, which is subject to the limitations discussed in Chapter 4, is shown in Table 6.3. It is apparent that the statistical power of one of the endpoints was less than 80 per cent even for a test drug outcome of 100 per cent success! Only one endpoint had 80 per cent power to detect a differential between test and control of 10 per cent, whilst two endpoints had 80 per cent power to detect only very large differentials above 50 per cent. It follows that, for all but one of these endpoints, there was a substantial chance of missing a sizeable benefit for the test drug. Calculations were not performed for two trials with quantitative endpoints (Reilly *et al.* 1986; Weimar *et al.* 1980) for the reasons set out in Chapter 4. However, both trials were very small (6 *versus* 7 and 8 *versus* 8 patients, respectively) and so the statistical power of both was undoubtedly very low.

Table 6.3 Statistical power calculations

Test drug	Control group	Smallest patient group	Control success	Measure of success	Per cent test drug success for 80 per cent power	Test-control differential for 80 per cent power	Reference
α IFN	PBO	6	33.3	No subepithelial infiltration	94	61	Adams *et al.* (1984)
β IFN	PBO	11	18.2	Disappearance of warts	69.2	51	Schonfeld *et al.* (1984)
LEVA	PBO	81	89.4	No major postop. infection	99.4	10	Ausobsky *et al.* (1982)
		81	97.4	Survival	impossible	—	

Almost none of the trial reports included a patient reject log (question 14). Winston *et al.* (1982) reported that, of a consecutive series of 68 presentations for bone marrow transplantation, 14 were rejected from trial participation: 5 were undergoing syngeneic transplantation from an identical twin (the patient selection criteria specified allogeneic transplantation), 8 had a pre-transplant anti-CMV titre outside specified limits and one had a prior positive urine culture for CMV.

Rather few of the studies surveyed gave details of the general state of health of the patients (question 16). In a study of adenovirus kerato-conjunctivitis, Reilly *et al.* (1986) excluded patients with systemic or other viral diseases. A particular concern with any trial of immunomodulators is the possible confounding effect of the AIDS virus, HIV. This is an especial problem in trials on hepatitis B in homosexual patients, and it would help with the comparison of results between studies if the trialists would state their policy on enrolment of HIV patients. Perrillo *et al.* (1988) excluded 'patients with HIV with clinical manifestations of AIDS or related syndromes. Asymptomatic male homosexuals with a positive test for antibody to HIV were not specifically excluded'. Studies with patients with sepsis or who were drug abusers automatically scored '0' for question 16 as explained in Chapter 4.

Regarding adverse immunological events (question 25), most of the interferon studies paid special attention to the development of leuco-paenia, especially during the first few weeks of therapy. Four of the trials included in this survey were conducted upon transplant recipients at risk of CMV reactivation. Trials of immunomodulators in transplant patients present a unique situation in which the need to stimulate an immune response against the infectious agent is tempered by the need to avoid provoking rejection of the graft or, in the case of bone marrow transplants, graft-versus-host disease. A further potential problem arises from an incomplete understanding of the processes whereby leucocytes escape from normal developmental control, resulting in leukaemia. Some immunotherapeutic agents are potent modulators of cellular growth and differentiation and may influence the underlying disease process in leukaemic patients as well as having an effect upon the target infections. Relevant information was provided in some studies. For example, Winston *et al.* (1982), in a study of a hyperimmune anti-CMV preparation in patients receiving bone marrow, tabulated deaths according to whether they were caused by interstitial pneumonia (trial efficacy endpoint), graft-versus-host disease or leukaemic relapse. Hirsch *et al.* (1983) used interferon in renal transplant patients and reported that 'survival of patients and grafts was equivalent in both treatment groups'.

Other questions which usually achieved a low score according to the criteria in Chapter 4 were: statistical reporting (question 31), reporting of interruptions to drug administration (question 19), exclusion of concomitant therapies (question 20) and the reporting and analysis of censorship (question 30).

QC questions   None of the trials reported data auditing or tests for blindness. None of the multicentre trials in which laboratory variables were monitored mentioned QC testing of the effects of transportation upon laboratory samples. Measures to assure or check on compliance for self-administered drugs were mentioned. In a study of an intranasal interferon preparation as a prophylactic for natural rhinovirus infection amongst office workers (Farr *et al.* 1984), a study nurse supervised administration of the nasal spray for the weekday doses, although the weekend doses were unsupervised. Reilly *et al.* (1986) rejected five patients from a study of interferon eyedrops for adenovirus conjunctivitis because of lack of compliance.

NRCTs

The scores achieved by the 17 NRCTs ranged from 27 to 70 per cent, with a mean of 52.6 per cent and a median of 55 per cent. There was no correlation ($R^2 = 0.14$) between score and year of publication, which ranged from 1980 to 1989. Five of the NRCTs were performed on AIDS patients and these are also considered on p. 140.

Table 6.4 shows which questions most frequently achieved each possible score. The pattern is very similar to that obtained for RCTs on patients with infections. Most studies described a series of patients rather than a set of selection criteria (question 9). Smaller patient numbers and tabulation of individual patient data ensured that information about losses to follow-up was usually available (question 27).

Of seven comparative NRCTs, one used historical controls (Meyers *et al.* 1980), one used a composite of historical controls and persons who refused to participate actively in the trial (Beasley *et al.* 1983), three used age and sex matched patients (Palmisano *et al.* 1988; Scott *et al.* 1980; Higgins *et al.* 1983), one had a single placebo recipient (Marget *et al.* 1985) and one used patients who did not meet an inclusion criterion for the active treatment group (Palmovic 1987). In the last case, healthcare workers who presented within 3 days of needlestick or permucosal exposure to Hepatitis B were immunized whilst those presenting after 3 days served as controls. The two groups were therefore not comparable. At the very least there needs to be an upper limit on the time since exposure for eligibility for the control

Table 6.4 Score frequencies for each question for the infection NRCTs

Question number	Subject of question	Score frequency (per cent)			Sample* number
		2	1	0	
Questions which usually scored '2':					
1	Number of endpoints	42.86	14.29	42.86	7
2	Definition of endpoints	53.33	13.33	33.33	15
3	Blindness of patients to treatment	50.00	0.00	50.00	6
4	Blindness of clinicians to treatment	50.00	0.00	50.00	6
6	Choice of statistical methods	33.33	33.33	33.33	9
10	Reporting of patient numbers	100.00	0.00	0.00	17
12	Patient withdrawal log	71.43	0.00	28.57	7
14	Reporting of dosage regimen	88.24	11.76	0.00	17
19	Objectivity of clinical monitoring	94.12	5.88	0.00	17
24	Reporting of baseline patient data	76.47	11.76	11.76	17
25	Reporting of results	76.47	17.65	5.88	17
27	Analysis of dropouts	58.33	8.33	33.33	12
Questions which usually scored '1':					
9	Reporting of patient selection criteria	47.06	52.94	0.00	17
20	Relevance of immunological monitoring	30.77	61.54	7.69	13
21	Close monitoring for adverse events	29.41	35.29	35.29	17
26	Adverse event reporting	35.29	47.06	17.65	17
28	Statistical reporting	22.22	44.44	33.33	9
Questions which usually scored '0':					
5	Blindness to ongoing results	0.00	0.00	100.00	6
7	Homogeneity check on multicentre data	16.67	16.67	66.67	6
8	Trial size	5.88	0.00	94.12	17
11	Patient reject log	0.00	6.25	93.75	16
13	Exclusion of concomitant diseases	11.76	5.88	82.35	17
15	Identity of comparator in blind studies	33.33	0.00	66.67	3
16	Interruptions to drug administration	6.25	25.00	68.75	16
17	Exclusion of concomitant therapies	11.76	11.76	76.47	17
22	Adverse immunological event reporting	5.88	41.18	52.94	17
23	Uniformity of multicentre evaluations	0.00	33.33	66.67	3
Questions which were 'NA' in every case:					
18	length of washout in crossover studies				

*Sample number = the number of trials scored minus the number for which the question was not applicable

group, otherwise the disease could have already established before immunization was commenced. Beasley *et al*. (1983) gave reasons for believing that bias would not be introduced by the use of non-randomized controls. Firstly, the primary endpoint—HBsAg carrier state—was determined by laboratory staff who were blind to whether or not the child had received vaccination. Secondly, the rate of acquisition of the carrier state had been very consistent for 10 years and could be expected to be the same in two groups of participants whether those groups were obtained by randomization or not. Two of the studies employing age and sex matched controls were trials of interferon for prophylaxis of the common cold (Scott *et al*. 1980; Higgins *et al*. 1983). Both studies used a placebo for the control group, blindness presumably being achieved by having one member of staff perform the matching and treatment allocation and another perform the administration and assessment.

As regards the QC questions, two trials mentioned estimating compliance by counts of empty containers (Smith *et al*. 1982) or weighing nasal spray containers (Higgins *et al*. 1983). Carter *et al*. (1987) provided the only example of data auditing encountered during the entire survey of 190 clinical papers reported in this book. The trialists state: 'At the termination of the study an independent field audit of the clinical and laboratory data . . . was also conducted . . . which concluded that the data are an accurate presentation of that generated during the course of the study'.

Special features of AIDS trials

Eleven AIDS trials have been included in this survey. Four considered only or principally the effects of therapy upon Kaposi sarcoma—the scores achieved by these studies (1 RCT and 3 NRCT) were reviewed in the cancer section (chapter 5). Seven considered the more general aspects of the disease—the scores achieved by these studies (2 RCT and 5 NRCT) were included in the present chapter.

Studies of Human Immunodeficiency Virus (HIV) infection present the clinical trialist with a number of special problems, whether the drug be an immunotherapeutic agent or an inhibitor of viral activities such as AZT (azido-deoxythymidine), DDI (dideoxyinosine) or the 'sugar mimics' being developed by Organon, Merrel–Dow and Monsanto–Searle which interfere with the attachment of HIV to the T-lymphocyte (BBC 1990).

The acquisition of HIV infection is an emotive event and patients often feel reluctant to enter trials in which there is a 50/50 chance of their receiving a placebo rather than active treatment. One way around this problem is to offer patients the choice of participation in either of two concurrent randomized trials, one of which includes a placebo group and one of which does not. This strategy has been adopted by the current international trial of DDI coordinated by Britain and France (Anon 1990). In one trial, patients will be assigned at random to receive either high dose DDI, low dose DDI or placebo. In the other trial, patients will be randomized to high or low dose DDI only. It will be interesting to see what proportion of patients opt for the placebo-controlled trial and whether any observed benefit for high dose (compared to low dose) DDI in the two studies is comparable. Another way of ensuring that all patients receive active treatment in a comparative trial is to cross over the control patients to the active treatment at the end of the observation period. However, this strategy is limited to short term studies as illustrated by the Imuthiol trial (Lang *et al.* 1988).

The clinical course of HIV infection can be lengthy and trials with endpoints such as death or clinical deterioration, whilst ultimately the most rigorous and clinically meaningful test, can be cumbersome. Problems of loss to follow-up and compliance can be considerable, particularly if another potential but unproven treatment becomes available which in the popular imagination is regarded as a better option than the trial drug. These problems can only increase as the disease drifts through the socio-economic groups, giving a greater proportion of poorly-educated, drug-abusing prostitutes and a smaller proportion of educated, affluent persons as appears to be happening in San Francisco. Checks on compliance with the dosage regimen (e.g. counting of remaining pills) should be performed routinely, backed up by blood levels to confirm that the patient is not simply discarding the requisite number of pills prior to a follow-up visit. This presupposes the availability of facilities for handling of HIV positive blood samples at the follow-up clinics.

If loss to follow-up, lack of compliance and resistance to placebo-controlled trials become severely limiting, then the rather unpleasant implication is that there will be a kind of natural selection of the best available therapy: any patients, currently infected, who are still alive in twenty years will be those who, by moving from trial to trial at whim, chanced upon the right treatment, leaving in their wake a stalled rational drug selection programme. A cure for AIDS *will* ultimately be recognized—as evolution takes its course.

In an attempt to manage the situation, the American Food and Drug Administration (FDA) is currently reviewing the whole field of AIDS trials and early (pre-trial) availability of experimental treatments under its 'compassionate use' mechanism (Vaughan 1990). Whilst 'patients' rights' groups are pressing for early release of potential new drugs, the FDA has also to weigh the daunting ethical and liability implications. On the one hand, is it right to withhold a treatment that a patient with a progressive and ultimately lethal condition wants to try, in favour of a slow and (as the patient sees it) unnecessarily bureaucratic process? On the other hand, the whole realm of anti-viral (let alone anti-retroviral) drugs and immunomodulatory agents is a new one and perhaps fraught with unpredictable (perhaps awful) side-effects that would only reduce the quality of the patient's remaining lifespan. Alternatively, should it be viewed as fortunate that on this rare occasion there are so many volunteers available for phase one studies of new drugs? Rather unhelpfully, one 'patients' rights' group has threatened to sabotage clinical trials of new AIDS drugs unless they are made more widely available. There seem to be two ways out of this situation which the FDA are considering. Firstly, trials could be run in parallel with a greatly expanded compassionate availability, so that rigorous testing would continue but all patients outside the trial would also have access to the drug. The other is to run very large clinical trials, enrolling every AIDS patient. Such studies would have a small number of simple endpoints, enabling monitoring to be performed at the GP level.

There is clearly a need for more convenient, rapidly evaluable endpoints such as a cell count or an antigen titre which is predictive of clinical outcome. Persistence of HIV antigens (e.g. p24), for example, has been associated with increased risk of progression (de Wolf *et al.* 1987 and Moss 1988). Following reports that p24 antigenaemia could be suppressed by AZT (*in vivo*) and alpha- or beta-interferon (*in vitro*), Orholm *et al.* (1989) attempted combined low dose therapy in a series of 12 patients who were asymptomatic or had persistent generalized lymphadenopathy (PGL). Avoidance of toxicity (due to AZT or the high doses of interferon predicted by the *in vitro* work) provided the rationale for the study, synergism of the two drugs having been noted *in vitro*. A statistically significant reduction in p24 titre was observed using AZT doses of up to 800 mg/day and interferon doses of up to 3×10^6 IU/day, four patients requiring reduction of AZT dosage and three receiving transfusions. The clinical relevance of this observation can be investigated in larger, controlled trials in which the long term clinical outcome is monitored as well as the short term changes in antigenaemia in order to determine whether or not modification of p24 levels does indeed modify the clinical course. Kovacs *et al.* (1989) also observed a loss of p24 antigenaemia, in three of six patients, using a combined interferon and AZT regimen. de Wit *et al.* (1988), in a trial on full-blown AIDS patients with Kaposi sarcoma, provided confirmation that high dose interferon (up to 36×10^6 IU on day 4 attained by an escalating regimen) can reduce HIV-antigen titre. Significantly, this reduction was seen predominantly in those patients whose tumours regressed and the trialists report that 'objective toxicity was slight or absent'. Jackson *et al.* (1988) investigated the effects of hyperimmune anti-p24 serum in six patients with AIDS or severe ARC and observed a reduced symptom score, increased Karnofsky index and a tendency towards weight gain during the 4–11 weeks of freedom from antigenaemia conferred by passive immunization.

Carter *et al.* (1987) used nucleic acid hybridization techniques to monitor levels of HIV-RNA in peripheral blood mononuclear cells (PBMC) following their dissolution with guanidine thiocyanate. However, neither the RNA level nor the HIV load (estimated by co-culture of patients' PBMC with PHA-stimulated normal PBMC) correlated with the titre of HIV antigen (described as 'mainly p24' by the trialists) at baseline. Indeed several patients were RNA positive and p24 negative. Carter *et al.* (1987) obtained, using a double-stranded RNA preparation ('Ampligen'), a rapid fall in HIV-RNA levels preceding a fall in HIV-antigen titres, although the number of patients was small.

The presentation of HIV infection is heterogeneous, patients being grouped under headings such as 'AIDS related complex (ARC)', 'lymphadenopathy syndrome' or 'full-blown AIDS', each with its own constellation of symptoms and signs. Infected persons may also be asymptomatic. It is therefore important that trialists specify precisely what sort of patients were enrolled to enable meaningful comparisons to be drawn between studies. The American Centers for Disease Control have published criteria for defining the various stages of HIV infection (CDC 1986).

It is equally important to specify which of the various features of the disease were being monitored as the primary endpoint. It is quite unacceptable to refer to patients simply as 'clinically improved' without stating which symptom or sign improved, according to which monitoring technique and the magnitude of the improvement. The multifaceted nature of the disease suggests the use in clinical trials of an index of clinical improvement encompassing several features of the disease, although indices with true clinical importance rather than just anecdotal value are not easy to derive, especially when long term follow-up may be confounded.

External, blinded monitoring committees also have a role in objectively assessing the varied and complex patient data for overall treatment success or failure. Such committees could use sequential statistical methods, with stopping rules specified at the outset in AIDS trials with long term clinical endpoints (e.g. death or progression to full blown AIDS) to ensure that significant results are recognized as early as possible but without sacrificing statistical safeguards.

Groopman *et al.* (1987) pointed out the difficulty of distinguishing adverse events from the wide range of symptoms and signs arising from the complex natural history of the disease itself. Detection of adverse events is further confounded in trials on drug abusers by the effects of their addiction.

Finally, the drug may induce further unwanted immunological effects [questions 24 (RCT) and 22 (NRCT)] such as the well known myelotoxicity of AZT or more complicated immunomodulatory effects.

As Chapter 1 makes clear, the immune system is a complex network of cells and soluble mediators. In the normal system, an antigenic challenge is recognized by a range of specific and non-specific 'sensors' (B lymphocytes, T lymphocytes, NK cells, monocytes, etc.) and numerous 'effector' pathways can be activated (T cell or NK cell cytotoxicity, complement, phagocytosis, antibody-dependent cellular cytotoxicity, etc.). Numerous, inter-related 'processors' mediate the flow of information and instructions between sensors and effectors. There are also mechanisms by which tolerance is maintained towards self antigens or can be induced towards certain foreign antigens.

In AIDS, this network has been severely perturbed by the HIV, resulting in immunosuppression and a predisposition to opportunistic infection and Kaposi sarcoma. There has even been a suggestion of autoimmune damage to the thymus epithelium (Savino *et al.* 1986), although a specific anti-thymic antibody has not been identified. To this altered and still not fully characterized baseline is then added a second perturbation in the form of an immunomodulatory drug which brings about a further constellation of changes, not all well characterized, within the immune system. It would be an act of unimaginable serendipity if the perturbation induced by the immunomodulator precisely cancelled that resulting from HIV infection. The immune system will more likely enter a third state which differs from either the normal state or the HIV infected state. Whether or not this new state is beneficial to the patient will depend upon whether it favours or hinders HIV, can maintain self-tolerance and can assume the normal role of protecting the patient against infection and cancer. Short term trials may demonstrate a helpful reconstituion of cell numbers, but the revitalized immune system may later be found to have undesirable properties.

Palmisano *et al.* (1988) discussed the possibility of a thymus hormone preparation increasing the number of viral targets by stimulating CD4 expression and activating CD4+ cells. By 'feeding the virus' in this way it is conceivable that these agents could worsen the disease. However, more clinical deterioration was observed during an 18-month observation period in the control group (3 of 24 progressed from ARC to AIDS) than amongst the thymus hormone recipients (0 of 34 progressed from ARC to AIDS) and the trialists point out that only a small proportion of the available *in vivo* T-cell population appears to be infected with HIV (Klatzmann and Gluckman 1986), suggesting that the virus would not necessarily take advantage of a further supply of T-cells. However, the sample number for the progression observations is low and could represent chance variation. To attempt to prove, in a fresh trial, that fewer patients progressed to AIDS when in receipt of thymus hormone, with a placebo success rate of 87.5 per cent (21 of 24 control patients did not progress to AIDS), at least 106 patients would be required per treatment group to have at least an 80 per cent chance of detecting as significant (at the 5 per cent level) an improvement of this figure to 97.5 per cent for the active treatment.

Trials routinely included monitoring of white cell counts, although it may be difficult to ascribe any worsening of counts to, for example, the transient myelosuppression associated with interferon rather than to the natural history of the HIV infection. The incidence of autoimmune diseases, allergic reactions, cancer, or the rejection of pre-existing grafts which had been tolerated before receipt of the immunotherapeutic agent should be monitored in the long term to determine the suitability of the new state of the immune system. Laboratory tests for some well known autoantibodies could be performed as part of short term viral marker trials.

Mechanism of action of 'high-score' agents

Amongst the 55 trials included in this survey of immunointervention in infectious disease, 'high score' status was achieved by studies of interferon as well as both active and passive immunization.

The phenomenon of immunological memory is the most extensively exploited feature of the immune system, although much remains to be learnt about the mechanism by which it operates. It is thought that when B lymphocytes are stimulated to proliferate by antigen, a small proportion of them do not proceed all the way to fully-differentiated antibody-producing cells. Instead they re-enter a dormant phase of the cell cycle awaiting a second stimulation by antigen. That memory cells are different from the original unstimulated B cell population is indicated by their ability to respond to antigen more rapidly and in lower concentrations. Passive immunization, with specific immunoglobulin, is a convenient means for providing cover whilst endogenous antibody production gets underway, particularly when slow primary responses are involved.

The possible mechanisms for the anti-viral action of interferons have been reviewed recently (Pestka *et al.* 1987 and Stanton *et al.* 1987). As well as a wide range of effects upon the activity of cellular components of the immune system, interferons modulate the activity of several intracellular enzymes which can interfere with protein synthesis. The best known of these are 2'5'-oligoadenylate synthetase and P1/eIF2, a protein kinase, both of which are induced by interferons and are active only in the presence of double-stranded RNA, such as that carried by some viruses. However, the precise quantitative contribution of such mechanisms *in vivo* is unclear and the numerous other actions of interferons, as well as the wide range of viruses against which interferons can act, cloud the picture.

Appendix 6.1: List of randomized trials of vaccines included in this survey

Test drug	Test patients evaluated	Control treatment	Control patients evaluated	Outcome of scoring	Reference
CHOLERA KWC+B−TOX	20705				
CHOLERA KWC	20743	PBO	20837	GA	Clemens et al. (1988)
JAP ENCEPH 2 STRAIN	22080				
JAP ENCEPH 1 STRAIN	21628	PBO	21516	GA	Hoke et al. (1988)
BOV ROTA + POLIO(o)	78				
BOV ROTA + POLIO(iM)	92	PBO + POLIO(o)	91	GA	Hanlon et al. (1987)
SIMIAN ROTA	123	PBO	124	GA	Flores et al. (1987)
BOV ROTA	86	PBO	92	GA	Vesikari et al. (1984)
BOV ROTA	168	PBO	160	GA	Vesikari et al. (1985)
CMV	53	PBO	38	GA	Plotkin et al. (1984)
LEISHMANIA	1325	PBO	1261	GA	Antunes et al. (1986)
HEPATITIS	442	PBO	423	GA	Szmuness et al. (1982)
HEPATITIS	714	PBO	688	GA	Francis et al. (1982)
HEPATITIS	184	PBO	170	HS	Crosnier et al. (1981)
HEPATITIS	285	TET−DIPTH+POL	241	GA	Maupas et al. (1981)
HEPATITIS	397	PBO	403	GA	Coutinho et al. (1983)
HEPATITIS	549	PBO	534	GA	Szmuness et al. (1980)
HEPATITIS	35				
HEPATITIS + HBIg(LD)	33				
HEPATITIS + HBIg(HD)	35	PBO	34	HS	Wong et al. (1984)

Appendix 6.2:   **List of randomized trials of immunological agents for infectious disease included in this survey**

Test drug	Test patients evaluated	Control treatment	Control patients evaluated	Nature of infection	Purpose of trial	Outcome of scoring	Reference
α IFN	21	PBO	18	Varicella zoster	T	GA	Arvin et al. (1982)
α IFN	125	PBO	132	Papillomavirus	T	GA	Eron et al. (1986)
α IFN	8	PBO	6	Adenovirus	T	GA	Adams et al. (1984)
α IFN	19	PBO	22	Rhinovirus	P	GA	Scott et al. (1982)
α IFN	8	PBO	8	Hepatitis B	T	GA	Weimar et al. (1980)
α IFN	20	PBO	22	Cytomegalovirus	P	HS	Hirsch et al. (1983)
α IFN	151	PBO	153	Rhinovirus	P	GA	Farr et al. (1984)
α IFN + PRED	18	none	21	Hepatitis B	T	GA	Perrillo et al. (1988)
β IFN	11	PBO	11	Papillomavirus	T	GA	Schonfeld et al. (1984)
β IFN	7	PBO	6	Adenovirus	T	GA	Reilly et al. (1986)
β IFN	10	IDU	10	Herpes simplex #	T	LS	Vannini et al. (1986)
PIS	17	NIS	18	Cytomegalovirus	P	GA	O'Reilly et al. (1983)
PIS	103	NIS	109	Septicaemia	T	GA	Ziegler et al. (1982)
PIS	24	none	24	Cytomegalovirus	P	GA	Winston et al. (1982)
PIS	30	none	32	Cytomegalovirus	P	GA	Meyers et al. (1983)
IgM enr Ig	30	PBO	30	Septicaemia	T	GA	Haque and Zaidi (1988)
ISOPRIN (LD)	16 }	PBO	30	Herpes simplex	T	GA	Salo and Lassus (1983)
ISOPRIN (HD)	15 }						
ISOPRIN	?	PBO	?	Herpes simplex	T	LS	Kalimo et al. (1983)
ISOPRIN + ACV	10 }	ACV	9	Varicella zoster	T	LS	Tanphaichitra and Srimuang (1987)
LEVA + ACV	12 }						
LEVA	81	PBO	85	Post-operative *	P	GA	Ausobsky et al. (1982)
TRANSFER F	16	PBO	15	Varicella zoster	P	GA	Steele et al. (1980)
IMUTHIOL	38	PBO	39	HIV	T	GA	Lang et al. (1988)
THYMOPENTIN	21	none	10	HIV	T	LS	Silvestris et al. (1989)

Appendix 6.3: List of non-randomized trials of immunological agents for infectious diseases included in this survey

Test drug	Test patients evaluated	Control treatment	Control patients evaluated	Nature of infection	Purpose of trial	Outcome of scoring	Reference
α IFN	7	None	12	Cytomegalovirus	T	GA	Meyers *et al.* (1980)
α IFN	35	PBO	35	Coronavirus	P	GA	Higgins *et al.* (1983)
α IFN	7	—	—	Papillomavirus	T	LS	Gibson and Harvey (1984)
α IFN	9	—	—	Hepatitis B	T	GA	Dooley *et al.* (1986)
α IFN	10	—	—	Papillomavirus	T	HS	Geffen *et al.* (1984)
α IFN + VID	7	—	—	Cytomegalovirus	T	GA	Meyers *et al.* (1982)
α IFN + VID	10	—	—	Hepatitis B	T	HS	Smith *et al.* (1982)
α IFN + AZT	11	—	—	HIV	T	GA	Orholm *et al.* (1989)
β IFN	15	PBO	14	Rhinovirus	P	GA	Scott *et al.* (1980)
HBIg+/−HBV	74	None	47	Hepatitis B	P	LS	Palmovic (1987)
HBIg+HBV	159	None	84	Hepatitis B	P	HS	Beasley *et al.* (1983)
PIS	6	PBO	1	Septicaemia	T	LS	Marget *et al.* (1985)
PIS	6	—	—	HIV	T	LS	Jackson *et al.* (1988)
IL-2	11	—	—	Hepatitis B	T	GA	Onji *et al.* (1987)
GM-CSF	16	—	—	HIV	T	GA	Groopman *et al.* (1987)
dsRNA	10	—	—	HIV	T	GA	Carter *et al.* (1987)
TP-1	34	None	22	HIV	T	LS	Palmisano *et al.* (1988)

Key to appendices to chapter six

Vaccines

CHOLERA KWC	killed whole cell cholera vaccine
CHOLERA B-TOX	B-subunit of cholera toxin
CMV	cytomegalovirus
HBV	hepatitis B vaccine
JAP ENCEPH	Japanese encephalitis virus
ROTA	rotavirus
(BOV ROTA	bovine rotavirus)
TET+DIPTH+POL	tetanus + diphtheria + polio vaccine

Other drugs

ACV	Acyclovir
αIFN	alpha-interferon (recombinant or leucocyte origin)
AZT	azido-deoxythymidine
βIFN	beta-interferon
dsRNA	double-stranded RNA ('Ampligen')
GM-CSF	granulocyte-macrophage colony stimulating factor
HBIg	hepatitis B immune globulin
IDU	iododesoxyuridine
IL-2	interleukin 2
IgM enr Ig	IgM enriched immunoglobulin
ISOPRIN	Isoprinosine
LEVA	Levamisole
NIS	non-immune serum
PBO	placebo
PIS	pooled immune serum or immunoglobulin
PRED	Prednisolone
TP-1	Thymostimulin
TRANSFER F	transfer factor
VID	Vidarabine

Purpose of trial

P	prophylactic
T	treatment of ongoing disease

Other

#	herpes simplex keratitis
*	infective complications following major laparotomy
(iM)	intramuscular route
(o)	oral route
HD	high dose
LD	low dose
HIV	human immunodeficiency virus

7

Immunosuppression of autoimmune and chronic inflammatory disorders

Introduction

Given the ability of the immune system to generate antibodies or T-lymphocyte receptors which are complementary to any antigen, the question arises as to how the immune system is prevented from attacking host tissues (Ehrlich's notion of 'horror autotoxicus'—see Himmelweit and Marquardt 1956). The mechanisms by which self-tolerance is maintained are the subject of much research, proposed mechanisms including clonal deletion, cell inactivation, and active suppression. New techniques, such as the generation of transgenic animals or monoclonal antibodies to T cell receptors of known, antigenic specificity, are yielding fresh insights (Crispe 1988). Immune complexes are also a common feature of many of these diseases, their dispersal in the blood causing inflammation at sites remote from the original pathogenic event.

In principle, there are as many autoimmune diseases as there are self-antigens for which tolerance can be lost and the clinical features of each disease will relate to the function of the organ(s) afflicted. Why some autoimmune diseases are far more common than others remains a mystery. Table 2.2 lists some of the commonest autoimmune and chronic inflammatory conditions.

As described in Chapter 2, current treatment involves, as a broad generalization, an initial attempt at inhibition of the inflammatory process using steroids and NSAIDs followed by the use of powerful, non-specific immunosuppressive drugs such as Azathioprine, Cyclophosphamide, or Methotrexate. In addition, several substances have been registered as anti-rheumatic agents: gold, penicillamine, chloroquine, and sulphasalazine. There remains, however, a significant proportion of patients who are resistant to these agents or who cannot tolerate the side effects. For example, the use of chloroquine can be limited by retinopathy and the use of gold carries the risk of dermatitis, renal toxicity, or myelosuppression. New approaches to the control of aberrant immunological processes are therefore required urgently.

In addition to suppression of the autoimmune or inflammatory onslaught, the treatment of these diseases requires the enhanced clearance of immune complexes. This simultaneous requirement for immunosuppression and immunostimulation provides one of the best examples of the true requirements of immunomodulation in clinical practice, and suggests that blanket immunosuppression by powerful cytotoxic agents will never provide the full answer. The use of plasmapheresis to remove circulating immune complexes has been reviewed recently (Jones 1985).

Special features of trials involving autoimmune and chronic inflammatory disorders

Several special features confront the trialist who ventures into the realm of autoimmune disease. These are listed below.

1. For some autoimmune conditions, such as rheumatoid arthritis (RA), there are numerous variables which can be monitored but no single variable provides an objective, unequivocal, universally acknowledged indicator of disease status (RCT questions 1, 2, and 22). The available methods for monitoring RA were reviewed recently by Furst (1988). They include subjective measures such as pain, duration of morning stiffness, and time to fatigue or more objective measures such as grip strength (measured by clasping a pressure gauge) and the number of tender or swollen joints. Several functional indices have been derived which involve the patient completing a questionnaire which asks questions about daily activities such as 'Can you reach up and get a 5 lb bag of flour from a shelf above your head?'. Examples include the Arthritis Impact Measurement Scale (AIMS) and the Health Assessment Questionnaire (HAQ). Given so many potential endpoints, attempts have been made to derive combined indices such as the Lansbury Systemic Index which combines morning stiffness, time to fatigue, pain medication usage, grip strength, and ESR (see p. 153). It is not easy to derive an index with clinical relevance rather than just anecdotal value, and considerable experience must be gained with indices in order to validate them. For clinical trials, the value of combined measures lies in reducing the number of endpoints for analysis in a clinical trial. Further, an index indicates an encouraging result only if several of the variables change favourably, thus avoiding the problem of interpreting the results in some trials where, for example, four of five variables, measured individually, show no difference between active and control treatments but one variable gives a highly significant result

in favour of the active treatment. The coefficient of variation (CV) has been determined for some of these endpoints by making repeat estimates in a series of 56 RA patients over a 1–2 week period during which time they underwent no change in medication. The CV, defined as the ratio of the standard deviation and the mean, ranged from 1.04 for morning stiffness to a mere 0.09 for grip strength. The Lansbury Systemic Index had a CV of 0.13 (Furst 1988).

Some autoimmune conditions are rather easier to monitor, having either a well established disability assessment scheme such as the Kurtzke (1965) scale for multiple sclerosis or a straightforward, quantitative, and clinically meaningful endpoint such as the insulin requirement in diabetics.

2. Nor is it always clear which immunological variables it is most useful to monitor (RCT question 23). In some autoimmune conditions (e.g. myasthenia gravis) a specific autoantibody has been demonstrated and monitoring of the production of this antibody provides a direct and relevant measure of immunological activity. No such discrete loss of self-tolerance has been observed for RA, however, and it is far less clear which immunological variables provide the most relevant information. Even the so-called 'rheumatoid factors' (anti-IgG) are found in patients with other diseases. Nor is the importance of these factors in the natural history of the disease known. Available methods for the laboratory evaluation of the rheumatoid and connective tissue diseases were reviewed recently by Morgan and Hughes (1985). The principal methods in routine use include erythrocyte sedimentation rate (ESR), C-reactive protein measurement (CRP), rheumatoid factor and anti-nuclear antibody titres, complement components, and immune complex determinations (ESR is related to the viscosity of the blood, which is altered by the presence of acute phase proteins; CRP is an acute phase protein). Morgan and Hughes state that 'ESR and CRP are of little use in differentiating RA from other inflammatory arthropathies, but in individual patients are good indicators of disease activity and response to treatment'.

A special feature of multiple sclerosis (MS) trials is the need to estimate immune reactivity in cerebrospinal fluid (CSF). An 'IgG index' is used, defined thus:

$$\text{IgG index} = \frac{\text{IgG in CSF}}{\text{IgG in serum}} \quad \text{divided by} \quad \frac{\text{albumen in CSF}}{\text{albumen in serum}}$$

If IgG is present in CSF because of a leak in the blood–brain barrier then the IgG index will be low because both IgG and albumen can leak through. If, however, the IgG is present due to synthesis in the CSF then the IgG index will be much higher. Agarose electrophoresis of the CSF from MS patients shows a characteristic pattern of IgG mobility known as 'oligoclonal bands'.

3. The importance of subjective endpoints for the evaluation of new drugs in certain chronic inflammatory conditions (e.g. RA) means that double-blind RCTs are essential (RCT questions 3, 4, 5, 6, 7, and 18). Large placebo effects may occur (Furst 1988), and results from non-controlled trials must be treated as very preliminary.

4. Many chronic inflammatory disorders follow a course of spontaneous exacerbation and remission. This makes it more difficult to determine efficacy than in conditions where the disease progresses steadily. Again, double-blind RCTs with well-matched groups of patients can help to distinguish spontaneous behaviour from treatment effect.

5. The rarity of some chronic inflammatory conditions may preclude the enrolment of sufficiently large numbers of patients (RCT questions 10, 11, 32).

6. Whilst criteria for diagnosis of the major autoimmune or chronic inflammatory conditions (e.g. RA or MS) are well established (American Rheumatism Association 1965, Ropes *et al*. 1958 and Ropes 1959 for RA; McDonald and Halliday 1977 and Poser *et al*. 1983 for MS) the patient population may be highly heterogeneous in terms of exacerbation frequency, level or nature of disability. The use of a wide spectrum of monitoring methods may reveal further baseline heterogeneity in terms of which variables are abnormal. Autoimmune conditions can occur in combination, such as pernicious anaemia with Hashimoto's disease or vasculitis with RA. Thus a trial of a drug aimed at one autoimmune disease may in fact only be tackling one part of a more complicated condition in some patients, whilst in others the disease may be uncomplicated by further autoimmune problems. Thus patient selection criteria must be clearly set out (RCT question 12), not least to allow comparisons to be accurately made between trials. The treatment groups must be carefully compared at baseline (RCT question 27) and the relationship of the selected group to the general population of patients with the disease should be indicated (RCT question 14).

7. Many immunosuppressive drugs have been associated with signi-

ficant adverse events (e.g. nephrotoxicity with Cyclosporin). Measures must be taken to allow for monitoring and responding to these events whilst maintaining blindness. It may be necessary to tailor dosage regimens according to individual patient responses. For example, a patient receiving Cyclosporin who develops nephrotoxicity will need dosage reduction. Some trials may employ an initially low dosage with an option of dosage escalation for those who show neither adverse nor beneficial responses. In such cases, published reports need to include information about the dosage modifications actually employed during the trial, otherwise comparison of the results from trials which nominally employed the same regimen may in fact not be comparing like with like.

8. It often may not be possible or ethical to withdraw ongoing symptomatic therapies during the trial, and so the study results will be obtained against a background of concomitant medication which could influence trial endpoints (RCT question 20). In such cases the aim should be to try to keep the consumption of concomitant medication stable and this should be substantiated by, for example, counting pills remaining from the previous prescription at each monitoring visit.

9. Immunosuppression could, in principle, give rise to infection and possibly even cancer in the long term. It is therefore especially necessary to monitor patients for adverse immunological events (RCT question 25—see Chapter 4).

Outcome of scoring

Forty trials comprising twenty RCTs (involving 996 evaluable patients) and twenty NRCTs (involving 1021 evaluable patients) were included in this survey.

RCTs

The scores achieved by the RCTs ranged from 26 to 70 per cent with a mean of 56 per cent and a median of 58.5 per cent. There was no correlation ($R^2 = 0.21$) between score and year of publication which ranged from 1980 to 1989. Seven of the studies were published in 1988, thus heavily biasing the distribution of year of publication. The scores amongst these seven studies ranged from 48 per cent to 70 per cent. Table 7.1 shows which questions most frequently achieved each possible score. For reasons of clarity, questions, 1, 2, 22, and 23, relating to

Table 7.1 Score distribution for RCTs

Question number	Subject of question	Score frequency (per cent) 2	1	0	Sample* number
Questions which usually scored '2'					
2	Definition of endpoints	75.00	5.00	20.00	20
3	Informed consent before randomization	90.00	5.00	5.00	20
5	Blindness of patients to treatment	85.00	0.00	15.00	20
8	Choice of statistical methods	50.00	44.44	5.56	18
12	Reporting of patient selection criteria	80.00	20.00	0.00	20
13	Reporting of patient numbers	85.00	15.00	0.00	20
15	Patient withdrawal log	90.00	10.00	0.00	14
16	Exclusion of concomitant diseases	50.00	25.00	25.00	20
17	Reporting of dosage regimen	75.00	25.00	0.00	20
21	Length of washout in crossover studies	50.00	50.00	0.00	2
22	Objectivity of clinical monitoring	55.00	40.00	5.00	20
23	Relevance of immunological monitoring	100.00	0.00	0.00	16
24	Close monitoring for adverse events	85.00	15.00	0.00	20
27	Baseline comparison of patients	85.00	10.00	5.00	20
28	Reporting of results	75.00	20.00	5.00	20
30	Dropout accounting	66.67	22.22	11.11	18
Questions which usually scored '1'					
6	Blindness of clinicians to treatment	40.00	50.00	10.00	20
20	Exclusion of concomitant therapies	10.00	85.00	5.00	20
29	Adverse event reporting	40.00	60.00	0.00	20
31	Statistical reporting	0.00	72.22	27.78	18
Questions which usually scored '0'					
1	Number of endpoints	15.00	0.00	85.00	20
4	Method of randomization	0.00	20.00	80.00	20
7	Blindness to ongoing results	10.00	5.00	85.00	20
9	Homogeneity check on multicentre data	20.00	0.00	80.00	10
10	Trial size by power calculation	10.00	0.00	90.00	20
11	Other reason for trial size	0.00	0.00	100.00	18
14	Patient reject log	0.00	5.00	95.00	20
18	Identity of comparator in blind studies	35.29	23.53	41.18	17
19	Interruptions to drug administration	15.00	15.00	70.00	20
25	Adverse immunological event reporting	30.00	25.00	45.00	20
26	Uniformity of multicentre evaluations	9.09	0.00	90.91	11
32	Results in terms of trial size	5.56	16.67	77.78	18

*Sample number = the number of trials scored minus the number for which the question was not applicable

Table 7.2 Use of clinical monitoring methods amongst ten trials of immunological agents in rheumatoid arthritis

Method	Per cent frequency of use ($n = 10$ trials)
Grip strength	100
Morning stiffness	100
Pain	100
Number and/or severity of swollen and/or tender joints*	100
Patient's global assessment	70
Clinician's global assessment	60
Proximal interphalangeal circumference (ring size)	40
Walking time	30
X-rays	30
Extra-articular nodules	30
Functional index:	
Lee	30
HAQ	20
Unspecified	10
Time to fatigue	10
Prednisone requirement	10

* Some studies specified the Ritchie articular index (Ritchie *et al.* 1968).

endpoints and monitoring (see p. 152 and 153) have been considered separately from the other questions.

Endpoints and monitoring

These are most conveniently discussed separately for RA and the other autoimmune diseases.

Rheumatoid arthritis trials Of the 20 RCTs surveyed, 10 involved RA patients. The endpoints were almost always clearly stated with scoring systems defined or published sources referred to (question 2). A very large number of clinical endpoints were evaluated (question 1) in these studies, as shown in Table 7.2. It follows that the number of clinical endpoints per trial was very large. Yocum *et al.* (1988), for example, had 16 clinical endpoints, not including variables such as ESR and rheumatoid factor which are discussed below. In only three trials, however, was an indication of priority given. Dougados *et al.* (1988) and Amor *et al.* (1987) regarded the global assessments by patient and clinician to be the principal endpoints, whilst Cannon *et al.* (1989) defined 'important improvement' in terms of at least a 50 per cent decrease in joint tenderness or swelling. These trialists, however, analysed this endpoint on no less than eight occasions, as permutations of: intention-to-treat or completers; outcome at 8 weeks or 12 weeks; tenderness or swelling scores. Several other clinical endpoints were also analysed. The potential for spurious significance with so many end-points is enormous. Indeed Cannon *et al.* (1989), were confronted with a set of results in which statistical significance was achieved only for swelling scores at 8 weeks [whether by intention-to-treat (105 patients) or analysis of completers (84 patients)]. Results at 12 weeks or for joint tenderness were not significant. Wisely the trialists counsel caution in interpreting the clinical significance of the results.

Radiological assessment of joints was used by three studies (Miller *et al.* 1980; van Rijthoven *et al.* 1986 and Kinsella *et al.* 1980). In van Rijthoven *et al.* (1986), no significant intra-group or inter-group changes were observed, even though six other variables improved significantly in the Cyclosporin group. Indeed the radiological score worsened from 105 to 115. Kinsella *et al.* (1980) observed radiological deterioration in the three Levamisole patients who improved by other criteria. Miller *et al.* (1980) commented that 'joint erosions were difficult to assess serially because of variations in radiographic technique and because of the advanced degree of changes present in many patients at baseline. However, there were no obvious changes discerned in erosions at either week 16 or week 32'. At week 16, a significant benefit for active treatment over placebo had been observed according to other variables.

None of the trials utilized a statistical method to cope with multiple endpoints (Pocock 1987) or utilized an index (e.g. Lansbury) which combines several clinical endpoints into a single overall measure. Only one trial (Amor *et al.* 1987) monitored the use of concomitant medication as an endpoint. Perhaps the careful monitoring of concomitant symptomatic medication could be used more widely as a day to day measure of subjective well-being.

The extensive validation required for a new index was well illustrated by Ritchie *et al.* (1968) for an articular (joint tenderness) index. Amongst the issues considered were: inter- and intra-observer variation, correlation with other clinical variables, the effects of analgesic medication and the means used to apply pressure to the joints in order to detect the degree of tenderness.

In the absence of an unequivocal and objective measure of disease status, the consensus appears to be to make the patient feel better, in terms of morning stiffness, pain and joint tenderness, backed up by semi-objective measures such as grip strength (question 22). Monitoring of changes in variables such as tenderness, swelling, and global well-being can best be achieved when a patient is assessed at each successive visit by the same investigator as was specified in five of the ten trial reports surveyed (these five scored '2', the remainder '1' or '0' depending on the objectivity of the primary endpoint). Two of the trials (Amor *et al.* 1987 and Kantharia *et al.* 1989) monitored patients at the same time of day on each occasion, one of them early in the morning (Amor *et al.* 1987). There is a need for new and better clinical endpoints, but until one becomes available, there is clearly scope for methodological improvement to firm up the use of existing endpoints.

A wide variety of immunological variables were monitored, as shown in Table 7.3. All ten studies scored '2' for question 23 for monitoring variables which can be regarded as relevant, if not definitive, in the absence of a clear disease marker.

An ideal laboratory marker would correlate with, or even predict, changes in clinical status. Table 7.4 lists the results obtained with the two most commonly used laboratory methods [erythrocyte sedimentation rate (ESR) and rheumatoid factor (RF)] together with the clinical outcomes for the ten RA trials. There appears to be no clear correlation, for the mean treatment group results, between clinical improvement and either ESR or RF.

Table 7.3 Use of laboratory monitoring methods amongst ten trials of immunological agents in rheumatoid arthritis

Variable	Per cent frequency of use ($n = 10$ trials)
ESR	100
Rheumatoid factor	90
Anti-nuclear/DNA antibodies	60
Serum immunoglobulins	40
C-reactive protein	40
Complement (total or components)	20
In vivo response to mitogen or antigen	20
Delayed hypersensitivity	20
CD4, CD8, etc.	20
In vivo antibody responses	10
Alpha-1 glycoprotein	10
T-suppressor activity	10

Table 7.4 Showing the clinical outcome and the results of two commonly used laboratory tests for ten trials of immunological agents in rheumatoid arthritis

Reference	Treatment	Extent of clinical benefit*	Laboratory results**	
			ESR	RF
Yocum et al. (1988)	Cyclosporin HD	16 variables improved	no change	'no sig. change'
	Cyclosporin LD	no change	'no sig. change'	'no sig. change'
van Rijthoven et al. (1986)	Cyclosporin	5/9 variables improved	trend -ve	ND
	Placebo	no change	increased	ND
Dougados et al. (1988)	Cyclosporin	(sig. more patients	no change	no change
	Placebo	improved on cyclosporin)	no change	no change
Veys et al. (1988)	Gamma-IFN	1/9 variables improved	no change	'no sig. change'
	Placebo	1/9 variables worsened	no change	'no sig. change'
Cannon et al. (1989)	Gamma-IFN	(equivocal benefit for	increased	no change
	Placebo	IFN over placebo)	increased	no change
Kinsella et al. (1980)	Levamisole	(3/4 patients improved)	(reduced†)	(no change‡)
	Placebo	(5/10 patients improved)	(increased†)	('no sig. change'†)

Miller *et al.* (1980)	Levamisole	6/6 variables improved	reduced	reduced
	Placebo	2/6 variables improved	no change	no change
Mowat and Mowat (1981)	Levamisole	7/7 variables improved	reduced	trend -ve
	D-Penicillamine	5/7 variables improved	no change	no change
Amor *et al.* (1987)	Nonathymulin HD Nonathymulin LD Placebo Nonathymulin VHD Placebo	('clinical improvement was not correlated with .... sedimentation rate or rheumatoid test ...')		
Kantharia *et al.* (1989)	TP-5	(2/4 variables sig. better on TP-5)	no change	no change
	Placebo		no change	no change

* Results quoted (except for those in brackets) are statistically significant changes from baseline for the group mean or median

** 'Increased' or 'reduced' refer to statistically significant changes from baseline for the group mean or median
'Trend -ve' refers to a non-significant decrease in value of the group mean or median
'No change' implies no trend apparent in the data
'No sig. change' is quoted from the text of papers in which numerical data not given

† Change observed in those who improved clinically (not statistically significant)

‡ 1 improved; 1 unchanged; 1 worsened

Of the other immunological monitoring methods used, Miller *et al.* (1980) observed a correlation between *in vitro* PHA response and clinical outcome in patients receiving Levamisole. The enhancement of PHA responsiveness was statistically significantly greater in patients who showed a moderate or marked clinical response than in those who had no or minimal responses.

The monitoring, by Amor *et al.* (1987), of suppressor T cell (Ts) activity on IgM production by B cells infected with EBV is especially interesting in terms of the suggestion that EBV may be an aetiological factor in RA (Lotz and Vaughan 1988). However, no significant change in the number of patients with normal or deficient Ts activity was observed either on placebo or Nonathymulin, even though there was a significant clinical improvement on active treatment. There was a suggestion, however, that the baseline level of Ts activity may be predictive of outcome on Nonathymulin. In the same study, Nonathymulin patients who showed a 'good' or 'very good' clinical response had a higher CD4/CD8 ratio during treatment (mean of four observations) than did those who had 'nil' or 'moderate' clinical responses.

Amongst the four trials in which C-reactive protein was monitored, a statistically significant reduction was seen in the Cyclosporin group but not in the placebo group by Dougados *et al.* (1988) and this observation correlated with the clinical outcome (14/26 treatment successes on Cyclosporin versus 2/26 on placebo). Similarly, Yocum *et al.* (1988) observed a statistically significant reduction in C-reactive protein level only in the high dose Cyclosporin group and this correlated with the incidence of clinical improvement. No change in C-reactive protein level was seen on gamma-interferon by Veys *et al.* (1988) where clinical improvement was less marked than in Yocum *et al.* (1988) or Dougados *et al.* (1988). Nor was there a statistically significant improvement in C-reactive protein level in Kantharia *et al.* (1989) (0.07 g/l at baseline; 0.05 g/l after 7 weeks on TP-5) in which the clinical improvement was less marked than in Yocum *et al.* (1988) although almost comparable with Dougados *et al.* (1988).

Of the remaining variables monitored in the ten RA trials, Dougados *et al.* (1988) observed a marked decrease in alpha-1 glycoprotein amongst the Cyclosporin recipients, with no change in the placebo group [median changes and 95 per cent confidence intervals: -0.37 (-0.54 to $+0.19$) g/l and 0.0 (-0.19 to $+0.12$) g/l respectively]. This correlated with the observation of 14/26 'good' or 'very good' clinical improvements in the Cyclosporin group and only 2/26 in the placebo group.

Clearly, an ideal laboratory marker must await a better understanding of the aetiology and pathogenesis of RA. In the meantime, it is probably best to regard the laboratory results as anecdotal only and not to base any therapeutic decisions for the whole treatment group on them. If an individual patient demonstrates a marked correlation between clinical improvement and a laboratory marker, preferably of a predictive nature, then laboratory data may be more useful in that instance.

Other indications For some of the indications, such as IgA nephropathy and insulin dependent diabetes mellitus (IDDM), objective endpoints were available—urinary protein content and metabolic variables (blood glucose, glycosylated haemoglobin, C-peptide, etc.), respectively. Most of the studies, however, employed a scoring system such as the Kurtzke scale (Kurtzke 1965) for multiple sclerosis, the PASI system (Frediksson and Petterson 1978) for psoriasis and the 'strength score' for myasthenia gravis (Tindall *et al.* 1987). Only one study referred, albeit ambiguously, to each patient being assessed serially by the same clinician and none referred to duplicate assessments in order to enhance the reliability of the results, although this may be impracticable with some of the more complex scoring systems. One of the psoriasis studies scored three lesions at each time point and analysed only the median scores in an attempt to avoid some of the natural variation in the data (Ellis *et al.* 1986).

Again, most of the trials had several endpoints although they were usually defined. Tindall *et al.* (1987) employed endpoints which would indicate failure early in the course of clinical deterioration (insufficiency in respiration with a forced vital capacity of less than 1200 ml or difficulty swallowing with frequent choking) so that patients would be denied the available alternative therapies for as short a time as possible. Some studies, such as Lai *et al.* (1988), performed repeated *p*-value calculations at successive timepoints (not advisable) whilst others made some attempt to limit the number of endpoints by specifying particular comparisons, for example, at 6 months, 12 months and the mean result for the visits over the first 6 months (Tindall *et al.* 1987).

In contrast to the difficult situation for the immunological monitoring of RA, some marked correlations between clinical and immunological endpoints were observed for myasthenia gravis and IgA nephropathy. In the former case (Tindall *et al.* 1987), at the 6-month endpoint, the correlation between 'strength score' and the log titre of antibodies against the acetylcholine receptor was statistically significant in both placebo and Cyclosporin groups (Spearman coefficient 0.8026; $p = 0.0165$ for the Cyclosporin group). In the IgA nephropathy study (Lai *et al.* 1988), a statistically significant reduction in proteinuria was observed in the Cyclosporin group at 3 months and this was accompanied by a statistically significant reduction in serum IgA concentration. By contrast, neither variable changed in the placebo group.

Ellis *et al.* (1986), in a trial of Cyclosporin in psoriasis, enumerated T-cells, monocytes, antigen presenting cells, and leukotriene B4 (LTB$_4$) levels in skin lesion biopsy specimens. The latter was measured because this substance enhances human keratinocyte proliferation, and elevated levels have previously been observed in the skin of psoriasis patients. A 64 per cent decrease in LTB$_4$ was observed after 7 days of Cyclosporin and this decrease was significantly different ($p = 0.015$) from the change in the placebo group. This correlated with a statistically significant clinical benefit for the Cyclosporin group seen at 4 weeks.

The IgG content of the CSF was monitored in the three multiple sclerosis studies. A correlation with clinical results was seen in Rudge *et al.* (1989). This study comprised two parallel trials conducted in London and Amsterdam. Statistically significant clinical benefit was observed in the former location only. Interestingly, therefore, in the London trial there was a significant fall in IgG index in the treated patients but not in the controls, whilst in the Amsterdam trial there was no significant difference in IgG index between the treatment and control groups. Conversely, Knobler *et al.* (1984) observed that 'IgG indexes fluctuated independently from clinical course'. Jacobs *et al.* (1982) had only one patient in the trial with an abnormal IgG level at baseline which normalised after one year on interferon. This patient improved clinically. Knobler *et al.* (1984) saw no significant changes in oligoclonal bands in serial CSF samples.

It follows from the above that the most frequent scores for questions 2, 22, and 23 was '2' and question 1 usually scored '0'.

Outcome of scoring for questions 3 to 21 and 24 to 32

Questions which usually scored '2'   The use of subjective measures requires the strict blinding of the trial, and all but one of the trials employed some degree of blindness (questions 3, 5, and 6). In many instances, patients were assessed by two investigators, one blind (efficacy monitor) and one not (toxicity monitor), in order that dosage modifications could be made in response to adverse events without unblinding the assessment of efficacy (hence question 6 usually scored '1' according to the criteria in Chapter 4). Methods for maintaining the blinding of patients during dosage modification included telling the patients, prior to the trial, that changes might be made in active or placebo dosages (Ellis *et al.* 1986) and making changes in the volume of placebo administered to mimic changes in the active treatment (van Rijthoven *et al.* 1986). In some studies, the toxicity monitor based his dosage change recommendations solely upon the blood level of the active drug and a laboratory test (e.g. creatinine level) and hence contact between the unblind assessor and the patient was avoided. However, this tactic has the disadvantage of the patient having to report adverse events to the blind assessor, who may then be able to guess the treatment allocation because of a characteristic pattern of side-effects.

The tactic of employing an independent clinician for blind assessment of efficacy was also used in two open trials in which the treatments were very different and blinding was therefore impossible (BenEzra *et al.* 1988 and Mowat and Mowat 1981). BenEzra *et al.* (1988) also specifically stated that informed consent was obtained without knowledge of treatment allocation (question 3). Cannon *et al.* (1989) administered Acetaminophen to counter the fever and myalgia associated with interferon treatment. This presumably helped maintain blindness by decreasing or removing these 'tell-tale' symptoms, but this tactic did require the clinically unnecessary administration of Acetaminophen to placebo recipients. The related questions of randomization method, code-breaking and comparator identity (questions 4, 7, and 18) usually scored '0' and are discussed below.

Several studies discussed the distribution of the data when specifying statistical techniques in the 'Methods' section (question 8). For example, Dougados *et al.* (1988) chose non-parametric tests because of the non-normal distribution of the data. Tindall *et al.* (1987) log transformed the anti-acetylcholine antibody titres in order to obtain normally distributed data.

The number of patients enrolled and evaluated, the reasons for withdrawal, the times of censorship, and a clear policy for inclusion or exclusion of data in the analysis were generally reported (questions 13, 15, and 30). For example, van Rijthoven *et al.* (1986) tabulated times and reasons for discontinuation and clearly indicated in the results tables whether the data referred to the total patient entry or to those who had completed 6 months in the trial. Several other trials performed analyses both of the total patient entry ('intention-to-treat') and of those who completed participation, including Cannon *et al.* (1989) and Amor *et al.* (1987). Tindall *et al.* (1987) tabulated individual results for all 20 patients in the trial in terms of three possible defined endpoints (treatment failure, safety, and protocol violation) and the times at which these endpoints were reached. Lai *et al.* (1988) simply stated that 'all patients completed the trial'.

For the majority of trials, the patient selection criteria (question 12) and the baseline comparison of the treatment groups (question 27) were clearly set out. Standard diagnostic criteria for RA (American Rheumatism Association 1965; Ropes *et al.* 1958; Ropes 1959) or MS (McDonald and Halliday 1977; Poser *et al.* 1983) were used. Several trials set limits on variables in order to enrol patients of a particular severity (see p. 154). These criteria varied between trials and this should be considered when drawing comparisons. For example, Kantharia *et al.* (1989) selected RA patients with six or more swollen joints and two or more of the following: nine or more joints painful or tender on movement or pressure; morning stiffness lasting at least 45 minutes; ESR of at least 20 mm/h. By contrast, Amor *et al.* (1987) selected those who satisfied at least three of the following: at least three joints with effusion or synovitis; morning stiffness of at least 60 minutes duration; ESR of at least 30 mm/h; Ritchie index of at least 10; Lee index of at least 5.

Most of the studies excluded a range of concomitant diseases (question 16). Patients with renal or hepatic disease were usually excluded from Cyclosporin trials and enrolment threshold values for laboratory tests of renal and hepatic function were often stated. Cancer, active infection, and hypertension were also frequent exclusions. Ellis *et al.* (1986) simply chose patients who were known to the trialists, were in generally good health and did not have impaired renal function. Van Joost *et al.* (1988) excluded alcoholics and drug abusers.

The use of Cyclosporin in patients with IgA nephropathy is interesting in the context of renal toxicity. In 10 of 12 patients, a reduction in proteinuria of at least 50 per cent was observed but this was accompanied by a steady rise in the plasma creatinine level (Lai *et al.* 1988). After cessation of Cyclosporin, the level of proteinuria immediately increased whilst the level of creatinine was back to baseline at 2 months post-cessation. The trialists concluded that long-term continuous Cyclosporin treatment of IgA nephropathy should be discouraged and its use in other glomerulonephritides requires cautious evaluation.

Most of the trials monitored laboratory variables and subjective symptoms as well as overt signs of adverse events (question 24). At each visit Kinsella *et al.* (1980) asked the patient: 'How are the tablets suiting you and have they caused any upset?' It is helpful to know how subjective symptoms were elicited from patients; some studies may report more or fewer adverse events simply because of the way information was sought from the patients. The reporting of adverse events, which usually scored '1', and unwanted immunological events, which usually scored '0', are discussed below.

The dosage regimen was usually well reported (question 17) and, for the Cyclosporin trials, usually involved options for increase or decrease of dosage according to blood levels or adverse events which were monitored by unblind clinicians who took no part in efficacy assessment.

There were two crossover studies, one evaluating Levamisole in RA (Miller *et al.* 1980) and the other alpha-interferon in MS (Knobler *et al.* 1984). Both considered the possibility of carry-over effects from one treatment phase to the next. For those patients in the former trial who received 16 weeks of Levamisole followed by 16 weeks of placebo, the trialists compared the clinical variables at weeks 16 and 32 and observed a substantial carry-over effect. Several variables were still improved at 32 weeks compared to week 0, and the trialists concluded that they could not pool the results from this group with those from the group who had received placebo between weeks 0 and 16. Knobler *et al.* (1984) employed a 6-month washout period between treatment phases in a comparison of interferon and placebo. Blood levels of interferon were monitored and it was only detected during the active treatment phases. Of course, this does not preclude the carry-over to the placebo phase of an effect initiated during the interferon phase. Curiously, patients did better when they received interferon in the second treatment phase (i.e. after placebo) rather than in the first phase. The trialists speculate that this could be because the patients recognized the change from placebo to active treatment and thus were expecting an improvement.

As was observed for the other therapeutic areas, the reporting of results was usually adequate (question 28).

Questions which usually scored '1' Most trials excluded patients who were receiving or had recently received treatments (question 20; see point 8 on p. 155) such as gold, penicillamine, or anti-malarials, although the washout period varied from, for example, one month (Yocum *et al.* 1988) to three months (Miller *et al.* 1980). Some trials excluded steroids (van Rijthoven *et al.* 1986) whilst others monitored their use as a part of clinical assessment (Amor *et al.* 1987). Several trials permitted concomitant usage of aspirin and other NSAIDs but required that the dosage be kept constant. Dougados *et al.* (1988) reported the daily dosages of prednisolone and NSAIDs in the two treatment groups during and prior to the trial. In general more information needs to be given on how closely the consumption was monitored, especially in out-patient studies. Rather few reports specifically excluded other immunomodulators, Dupre *et al.* (1988), for example, excluded Inosiplex and Levamisole, whilst Cannon *et al.* (1989) excluded Levamisole and TP-5. The range of permitted concomitant medication and the monitoring of its use remains a source of variation between studies which should be borne in mind when drawing comparisons.

Some adverse event reporting was very scanty (question 29), often concentrating on nephrotoxicity (e.g. Cyclosporin trials) but with more information needed on the severity and duration of other events. Statistical reporting suffered from the usual range of faults set out in Chapter 4. Question 6 (blindness of clinicians) was dealt with in the previous section.

Questions which usually scored '0'   Only two of the trials specifically stated that the trialists remained unaware of the trial results until after the last patient had been assessed (question 7). None gave a clear account of the method of randomization (question 4), there being just a passing reference to random number tables or sealed envelopes in a small number of reports. Rather few of the 17 reports of double or single blind studies mentioned the identity of active and control treatments (question 18). In six trials (3 Cyclosporin, 2 thymic hormone and 1 Levamisole) the two treatments were stated to be indistinguishable. In particular, Ellis *et al.* (1986) comments that both appearance and taste were the same for an oral preparation and its corresponding placebo.

Only three of the twenty trials gave a reason for the size of the trial. Two performed power caculations (Yocum *et al.* 1988 and Feutren *et al.* 1986). One trial, lacking both a power calculation and predetermined stopping rules, was stopped early when the trialists, who were not blind to treatment allocation, performed an analysis and found statistical significance (Tindall *et al.* 1987). This scored '0' for question 11. Only one of the trials which had not performed a power calculation at the outset did so *post hoc* (Cannon *et al.* 1989), whilst several acknowledged the small size of their sample or the need for larger confirmatory studies. Cannon *et al.* (1989) also discussed the possibility of *type 1* error, having performed no less than 38 inter-group comparisons and found only a few significant differences.

Of the 16 'high score' or 'grey area' RCTs which lacked power calculations, 4 ultimately showed no statistically significant difference in efficacy between treatments (Kinsella *et al.* 1980; Mowat and Mowat 1981; Knobler *et al.* 1984 and Veys *et al.* 1988). Two reports (Amor *et al.* 1987 and Rudge *et al.* 1989) each comprised the results of two parallel trials. In both cases a significant benefit was observed for one trial but not the other. In an attempt to probe the scope for type II statistical error (the probability of concluding that two treatments have the same efficacy when there is really a difference), power calculations were performed according to the method described in Chapter 4. The outcome, which is subject to the limitations discussed in Chapter 4, is shown in Table 7.5. Calculations were not performed for the three

Table 7.5 Statistical power calculations

Test drug	Control treatment	Smallest patient group	Control success	Measure of success	Per cent test drug success for 80 per cent power	Test-control differential for 80 per cent power	Reference
Cyclosporin (London)	PBO	21	42.86	no 1-point decline in Kurtzke at 6 mths	82	39.1	Rudge *et al.* (1989)
		21	52.38	no 1-point decline in Kurtzke at 12 mths	89	36.6	
		21	38.10	no 1-point decline in Kurtzke at 24 mths	78	39.9	
Cyclosporin (Amsterdam)	PBO	16	73.68	no 1-point decline in Kurtzke at 6 mths	impossible	–	
		16	63.16	no 1-point decline in Kurtzke at 12 mths	99	35.8	
		16	42.11	no 1-point decline in Kurtzke at 24 mths	85	42.9	
Levamisole	PBO	4	50	global clinical improvement at 6 mths	impossible	–	Kinsella *et al.* (1980)
Nonathymulin (HD)	PBO	16	17.65	global improvement	62	44.4	Amor *et al.* (1987)
Nonathymulin (LD)	PBO	16	17.65	global improvement	62	44.4	
Nonathymulin (VHD)	PBO	15	33.33	global improvement	79	45.7	

studies with quantitative endpoints (Mowat and Mowat 1981; Knobler *et al*. 1984; and Veys *et al*. 1988), but they were very small studies (the smallest patient group being 14, 12, and 11, respectively) and they would therefore have had low statistical power. Of the studies for which calculations were performed, the statistical power for two of the endpoints was less than 80 per cent even for a test drug outcome of 100 per cent success! All of the other endpoints had 80 per cent power to detect a differential between test and control of greater than 35 per cent. This is expecting rather a lot of the test drug. It follows that there was a substantial chance of missing a sizeable benefit for the test drug.

As has been observed for the other therapeutic areas, none of the studies gave an adequate account of the patients who presented but were rejected or prevented from participating (question 14—see p. 154). Nor were interruptions to drug administration or criteria for inclusion in analysis of those who missed doses reported routinely (question 19). Miller *et al*. (1980) stated that 14 of 20 patients completed the 16-week period at the dose of 150 mg Levamisole daily and for those who had temporary interruptions gave reasons and the duration of interruption. Tindall *et al*. (1987) defined protocol violation as failing to receive trial medication for more than 5 days. Rudge *et al*. (1989) performed an intention-to-treat analysis regardless of whether or not patients had received trial medication according to the protocol.

The search for and reporting of adverse immunological events varied greatly between the studies surveyed (question 25; see point 9 on p. 155). The incidence of infections was often reported, although sometimes their nature, severity and duration was not indicated. Miller *et al*. (1980) gave a detailed account of an infection in a patient receiving Levamisole who developed agranulocytosis. Feutren *et al*. (1986) actively sought lymphoproliferative disorders in a trial of Cyclosporin by isoelectrofocusing of serum. None were detected. Cannon *et al*. (1989) considered the possibility of an allergic reaction to recombinant gamma-interferon.

There were 11 multicentre trials among the 20 surveyed. Only two reported on the homogeneity of the data between centres. Dupre *et al*. (1988) report that there was 'no significant variation of treatment effect among the individual centres or between Canadian and European groups'. Rudge *et al*. (1989) reported separately the results obtained with Cyclosporin in MS at the two centres in London and Amsterdam. The results were markedly different with a benefit being observed in the former centre but not the latter. One possible explanation, suggested by the trialists, is the lower dosage received by the Amsterdam patients. Another, however, is the low level of statistical power in both

London and Amsterdam trials (see Table 7.5). One report of a multi-centre trial (van Joost *et al.* 1988) did not require an analysis of results by centre because the overall outcome was such that the results must have been the same at both centres (10/10 placebo failure; 1/10 active failure). Dupre *et al.* (1988) standardized estimates of glycosylated haemoglobin, which were measured by different methods in the European and Canadian centres, by exchanging samples (question 26). The correlation coefficient between paired values was 0.985.

QC questions   None of the reports mentioned auditing of case report forms. One (Rudge *et al.* 1989) tested the blindness of the patients but not the clinicians. The exchange of samples between European and Canadian monitoring laboratories (Dupre *et al.* 1988) effectively tested the transportation method for deterioration of samples, although it is not stated whether the same method was used between peripheral hospitals and each central laboratory as between the two central laboratories. Regarding compliance, most of the Cyclosporin studies and some of the interferon trials (e.g. Knobler *et al.* 1984) monitored blood levels. Ellis *et al.* (1986) assessed the amount of medication which had been removed from the bottle and chose patients who were known to the trialists as reliable. There were examples, unfortunately, of out-patient studies of oral therapies in which neither compliance nor blood levels were checked.

NRCTs

Twenty NRCTs involving 1021 evaluable patients were included in this survey. The scores achieved by the NRCTs ranged from 26 to 73 per cent with a mean of 50.32 per cent and a median of 51.25 per cent. There was no correlation ($R^2 = 0.03$) between score and year of publication which ranged from 1981 to 1988. Table 7.6 shows which questions most frequently achieved each possible score.

Four trials were comparative, three using historical controls (DuRant *et al.* 1982; Jones *et al.* 1982 and Assan *et al.* 1985) and one involving a crossover of just three patients amongst a total enrolment of ten (Sany *et al.* 1982). Jones *et al.* (1982) used a historical control group comprising combined data from three different sources. Information about the patients in each database were tabulated and possible deficiencies of each source were discussed. Life-table graphs were presented for each source and significant differences between the plots were discussed. One of the historical groups had a far worse survival probability than the other two. Two comparisons were therefore made

Table 7.6 Score distribution for NRCTs

Question number	Subject of question	Score frequency (per cent) 2	1	0	Sample* number
Questions which usually scored '2'					
2	Definition of endpoints	80.00	10.00	10.00	20
10	Reporting of patient numbers	95.00	5.00	0.00	20
12	Patient withdrawal log	77.78	0.00	22.22	9
14	Reporting of dosage regimen	75.00	25.00	0.00	20
19	Objectivity of clinical monitoring	70.00	10.00	20.00	20
20	Relevance of immunological monitoring	72.73	18.18	9.09	11
21	Close monitoring for adverse events	40.00	30.00	30.00	20
24	Reporting of baseline patient data	60.00	30.00	10.00	20
25	Reporting of results	65.00	30.00	5.00	20
26	Adverse event reporting	55.00	20.00	25.00	20
27	Dropout accounting	42.86	35.71	21.43	14
Questions which usually scored '1'					
1	Number of endpoints	0.00	50.00	50.00	4
9	Reporting of patient selection criteria	20.00	75.00	5.00	20
17	Exclusion of concomitant therapies	31.58	36.84	31.58	19
Questions which usually scored '0'					
6	Choice of statistical methods	18.18	27.27	54.55	11
7	Homogeneity check on multicentre data	0.00	0.00	100.00	7
8	Reason for trial size	0.00	5.00	95.00	20
11	Patient reject log	0.00	0.00	100.00	20
13	Exclusion of concomitant diseases	10.00	10.00	80.00	20
16	Interruptions to drug administration	5.00	10.00	85.00	20
22	Adverse immunological event reporting	25.00	35.00	40.00	20
23	Uniformity of multicentre evaluations	0.00	33.00	67.00	3
28	Statistical reporting	9.09	27.27	63.64	11

N.B. Questions 3, 4, 5 (blindness), 15 (identity of comparator) and 18 (length of washout in crossover trials) were applicable to just one study in which 3 of 10 patients received both treatments in a crossover fashion. Both treatments were gamma-globulin preparations, and were therefore presumably identical. The time between finishing one treatment and commencing the next was reported for each patient. Assessments were performed by a clinician who was blind to treatment allocation.

*Sample number = the number of trials scored minus the number for which the question was not applicable

to evaluate the active treatment. Firstly, the active group was compared with a composite of all three control groups together and then with a composite of the two historical groups with the best survival. Although historical controls cannot replace contemporary randomized controls in drug evaluation, the provision of this kind of information about the historical data sources facilitates critical assessment of the likely value of the active treatment.

The scores for the questions dealing with endpoints and monitoring were essentially the same as for the RCTs. (Note that the number of endpoints—question 1—was only considered for comparative trials.) The worst offenders were amongst the SLE trials of which there were four in this survey. Terms such as 'clinically apparent improvement' or 'significant improvement' or 'no improvement' were used in some SLE trials without definition or any indication of what monitoring method was being used or even what aspect of this multi-faceted disease had improved. SLE trials are needed in which a clear endpoint is stated at the outset. This could mean aiming at one facet of the disease per trial or constructing an index which includes scores for several aspects, the patient being regarded as a success if a threshold index value is reached. However, it is not easy to construct an index which has true clinical relevance as opposed to mere anecdotal value.

Some of the RA studies reported using the same investigator for repeat assessments, thus enhancing the consistency of the data (Weinblatt *et al.* 1987 and Sany *et al.* 1982). Several trials had clear quantitative endpoints such as platelet count in ITP patients. Assan *et al.* (1985), in a trial of Cyclosporin for diabetes, monitored the levels of anti-islet cell antibodies and anti-islet cell cytotoxicity. The latter declined in all patients who went into remission whilst no consistent trend was observed in specific antibody levels.

For patient selection (question 9), most reports simply described a series of patients and their baseline characteristics (question 24) rather than listing a set of inclusion and exclusion criteria as was usual for RCTs. SLE studies referred to the ARA criteria (Cohen *et al.* 1971 and Tan *et al.* 1982). Rather few gave information about the general health of the patients in terms of the exclusion of patients with concomitant diseases (question 13). None of the trials indicated how their population related to the general population (reject log—question 11) and none gave a reason for the size of the trial (question 8), giving ample scope for unintentional bias. The numbers of patients enrolled, reasons for withdrawal, and the information about drop-outs were usually reported (questions 10, 12, and 27), this being facilitated by the smaller number of patients in NRCTs.

The intended dosage regimen was usually clear (question 14) but less information was given about whether it was actually received or not in terms of interruptions (question 16). Imbach *et al.* (1981*a*) indicated the times of immunoglobulin injections on graphs of individual patient results. Weinblatt *et al.* (1987) checked patient compliance by 'bottle counts' of Cyclosporin (QC question iii). Most trials made some restrictions on concomitant medication (question 17).

Results were usually clearly reported (question 25), although there were the usual problems with statistical methods and reporting (questions 6 and 28) in terms of the criteria set out in Chapter 4. Adverse event reporting (questions 21, 22, and 26) usually included some comments about adverse immunological events. For example, Nussenblat *et al.* (1983*a*) stated that no neoplasms, angioedema, or depression of NK cell activity were observed in their trial of Cyclosporin in patients with uveitis. Isenberg *et al.* (1981) observed angioedema in some of their SLE patients receiving Cyclosporin but saw no bone marrow suppression. Newland *et al.* (1983) sought anti-allotype and anti-isotype antibodies in patients receiving high-dose intravenous immunoglobulin for autoimmune thrombocytopaenia.

There were seven multicentre trials but none gave details of patients and results by centre (question 7). Four had endpoints which were routine (platelet count), subject to normal hospital laboratory QC and therefore did not need standardization between centres (question 23). The remaining three studies used less definitive methods but standardization was not discussed in detail. For example, Jones *et al.* (1982) defined the time to death starting from the original date of diagnosis, prior to the trial. This retrospective diagnosis of subacute sclerosing panencephalitis (SSPE) was made in each case by the patient's own doctor based upon 'relatively consistent' clinical criteria.

Mechanism of action of 'high-score' agents

Evidence of efficacy was reported in trials which achieved 'high-score' status for Cyclosporin, high-dose IgG and Nonathymulin.

The mechanism of action of Cyclosporin was recently reviewed (Hess *et al.* 1988). The agent is non-lymphotoxic and appears to inhibit IL-2 production and the early stages of T cell activation. Cytotoxic T cell responses to transplantation antigens are particularly affected, whilst suppressor T cells are spared. A variable B cell sensitivity has been observed. *In vivo* antibody production to T cell dependent and T independent, type 1 antigens (e.g. DNP-Ficoll) is sensitive, whilst the T independent, type 2 response (e.g. hapten-LPS) is resistant to the effect of Cyclosporin. *In vitro*, Con-A stimulation is sensitive but LPS or IL-4 stimulation is not. Proteins with Cyclosporin binding properties have been observed—cyclophilin and calmodulin. Hess *et al.* (1988) point out that the story is far from complete, with several paradoxical observations including, for example, observations of an enhancement of prostaglandin and thromboxane synthesis and IgE production.

The mechanism of action of high dose IgG in ITP was discussed by Ben-Yehuda *et al.* (1988) and Newland *et al.* (1983). In the short term it is thought that the IgG competes with the autoantibody-coated platelets for Fc receptors on cells of the reticulo-endothelial system (RES). However, the benefit appears to last longer than the blockade of the RES and may therefore involve other mechanisms such as modulation of T-suppressor cells or an interaction with the idiotype network.

Nonathymulin, formerly called Factor Thymique Serique (FTS), is a nonapeptide possessing properties suggesting a role in extra-thymic development of T cells although, as a general rule, such 'thymic hormones' cannot completely replace the function of the thymus *in vivo*. Receptors for FTS have been observed on T cells. The precise mechanism responsible for bringing about clinical improvement in an autoimmune disease is unknown but the trialists speculate upon the possible modulation of suppressor T cell activity.

Appendix 7.1   **List of randomized trials of immunological agents for autoimmune disease included in this survey**

Test drug	Test patients evaluated	Control treatment	Control patients evaluated	Disease	Outcome of scoring	Reference
Cyclosporin	22	PBO	21	Multiple sclerosis	GA	Rudge et al. (1989)
Cyclosporin	16	PBO	19			
Cyclosporin	57	PBO	53	Insulin-dep. diabetes	GA	Feutren et al. (1986)
Cyclosporin	20	PBO	20	Myasthenia gravis	GA	Tindall et al. (1987)
Cyclosporin	10	PBO	10	Psoriasis	GA	van Joost et al. (1988)
Cyclosporin	20	PRED. or CHLORAMB.	19	Behcet's syndrome	GA	BenEzra et al. (1988)
Cyclosporin	12	PBO	12	IgA nephropathy	GA	Lai et al. (1988)
Cyclosporin	9	PBO	13	Rheumatoid arthritis	GA	van Rijthoven et al. (1986)
Cyclosporin (HD)	12	CYCLOSPORIN (LD)	13	Rheumatoid arthritis	GA	Yocum et al. (1988)
Cyclosporin	11	PBO	10	Psoriasis	GA	Ellis et al. (1986)
Cyclosporin	26	PBO	26	Rheumatoid arthritis	HS	Dougados et al. (1988)
Cyclosporin	93	PBO	94	Insulin-dep. diabetes	HS	Dupre et al. (1988)
α IFN	12	PBO	12	Multiple sclerosis	GA	Knobler et al. (1984)
β IFN	10	none	10	Multiple sclerosis	LS	Jacobs et al. (1982)
γ IFN	54	PBO	51	Rheumatoid arthritis	GA	Cannon et al. (1989)
γ IFN	13	PBO	11	Rheumatoid arthritis	GA	Veys et al. (1988)
Nonathymulin (HD)	14	PBO	15	Rheumatoid arthritis	HS	Amor et al. (1987)
Nonathymulin (LD)	15					
Nonathymulin (VHD)	12	PBO	12			
TP-5	35	PBO	39	Rheumatoid arthritis	GA	Kantharia et al. (1989)
Levamisole	4	PBO	10	Rheumatoid arthritis	GA	Kinsella et al. (1980)
Levamisole	14	D-PENICILLAMINE	17	Rheumatoid arthritis	GA	Mowat and Mowat (1981)
Levamisole	10	PBO	10	Rheumatoid arthritis	GA	Miller et al. (1980)

Appendix 7.2 List of non-randomized trials of immunological agents for autoimmune disease included in this survey

Test drug	Test patients evaluated	Control treatment	Control patients evaluated	Disease	Outcome of scoring	Reference
Cyclosporin	8	—	—	Uveitis	GA	Nussenblat et al. (1983a)
Cyclosporin	5	—	—	Syst. lupus erythematosus	LS	Isenberg et al. (1981)
Cyclosporin	12	None	44	Insulin-dep. diabetes	GA	Assan et al. (1985)
Cyclosporin	16	—	—	Uveitis	LS	Nussenblat et al. (1983b)
Cyclosporin	10	—	—	Syst. lupus erythematosus	LS	Feutren et al. (1987)
Cyclosporin	9	—	—	Rheumatoid arthritis	HS	Weinblatt et al. (1987)
γ IFN	30	—	—	Rheumatoid arthritis	GA	Schindler et al. (1988)
TP-1	6	—	—	Aplastic anaemia	LS	Giustolisi et al. (1983)
Levamisole	142	—	—	Rheumatoid arthritis	GA	Veys et al. (1981)
Isoprinosine	98	None	333	Subac. scler. pan enceph.	GA	Jones et al. (1982)
Isoprinosine	12	None	15	Subac. scler. pan enceph.	LS	DuRant et al. (1982)
Cyproterone	7	—	—	Syst. lupus erythematosus	GA	Jungers et al. (1985)
19nortestosterone	10	—	—	Syst. lupus erythematosus	LS	Hazelton et al. (1983)
Danazol	14	—	—	Idiop. thrombo. purpura	GA	Buelli et al. (1985)
Danazol	22	—	—	Idiop. thrombo. purpura	LS	Ahn et al. (1983)
IgG	25	—	—	Autoimmune thrombocytopaenia	GA	Newland et al. (1983)
IgG	13	—	—	Idiop. thrombo. purpura	GA	Imbach et al. (1981b)
IgG	6	—	—	Idiop. thrombo. purpura	HS	Imbach et al. (1981a)
IgG	177	—	—	Idiop. thrombo. purpura	LS	Uchino et al. (1984)
PEgG	10	RPgG	3	Rheumatoid arthritis	GA	Sany et al. (1982)

8

Allergy hyposensitization

Introduction

As explained in Chapter 2, allergy is the excessive, sometimes inappropriate expression of the inflammatory response to an antigen
(known as an 'allergen' in this context), the consequence of which will
lie somewhere on a spectrum extending from mild, temporary discom-
fort to death. The type I reaction commences within minutes of antigen
exposure, the precise symptoms depending upon the nature of the antigen and the site of administration. Cutaneous oedema with erythema
and pruritis may occur, involving only the superficial dermis (urticaria)
or extending to the deep dermis and subcutaneous or submucosal
regions (angioedema). Rhinitis is also a common response. In more
severe cases, bronchial constriction may occur accompanied by severe
hypotension. This acute life-threatening condition is known as anaphylactic shock, and must be treated immediately with adrenalin to counteract smooth muscle contraction, oxygen for hypoxia, intravenous
fluids to combat the hypovolaemia, and measures to maintain the
airway such as tracheal intubation.

The term 'anaphylaxis' was introduced in the early years of this
century by Richet and Portier as the opposite of 'prophylaxis'. In the
latter process, prior exposure to antigen confers protection, whereas
anaphylaxis was seen as the loss of protection after initial exposure.
Richet and Portier demonstrated that dogs could survive initial exposure to large doses of sea anemone toxin but died after secondary
exposure to very small quantities a few weeks later.

Inflammation is the complicated, multi-channel mechanism by which
the effectors of the immune system are brought to a site of antigen
penetration and are stimulated to destroy the pathogen to which the
antigen is attached. This process involves such mechanisms as modulation of regional vascular smooth muscle contraction (vasodilatation and
vasoconstriction) to give increased blood flow to the site at the expense
of other regions, increased capillary permeability to permit access of
immune effectors, chemotaxis of immune effector cells, and activation
of immune effectors at the site. These processes result in the character-

istic oedema and erythema at the site, whilst over-expression results in widespread smooth muscle contraction and capillary leakiness, leading to bronchoconstriction and hypotension. The destructive action of the inflammatory process can spill over to the adjacent host tissues, sometimes resulting in more damage than that caused by the provoking pathogen. The liver is stimulated to synthesize and release a range of plasma proteins which are thought to be involved in the maintenance and regulation of the inflammatory process. The appearance of these proteins in the blood is referred to as the 'acute phase response' the level of some of them (e.g. C-reactive protein) or their incidental effects (e.g. upon blood viscosity or erythrocyte sedimentation rate (ESR)) being used to monitor inflammation. Other systemic effects include fever, leucocytosis, and muscle proteolysis. The inflammatory process as a whole has been reviewed in detail by Movat (1985), whilst Whicher and Dieppe (1985) give a detailed account of the acute phase proteins.

The initial steps in understanding the mechanisms underlying inflammation were taken by Sir Henry Dale, who discovered that histamine mimics many of the effects of anaphylaxis and that uterine smooth muscle from antigen-sensitized animals contracts and releases histamine on re-exposure to antigen. Specific sensitivity could be conferred upon the uterus of a naive animal by serum from a sensitized animal. Mast cells were shown to be the source of histamine, sensitized cells undergoing dramatic degranulation upon exposure to antigen. Subsequently, a wide range of inflammatory mediators have been demonstrated such as the eicosanoids. These are produced principally by mast cells, basophils, and macrophages from membrane phospholipids. The action of phospholipases yields arachidonic acid which is then metabolized by either the cyclo-oxygenase pathway to yield prostaglandins (PGE2, PGI2 etc) and thromboxanes or by the lipo-oxygenase pathway to give the leukotrienes (LTB4, LTC4 etc.).

There are problems with both of the usual therapeutic strategies: avoidance of allergens and inhibition of inflammatory mediators. Avoidance may not be practicable (e.g. pollen allergy) and the inflammatory response is mediated by so many molecules and routes, the precise profile probably varying according to allergen, route of administration, and dose, that effective inhibition of the inflammatory process may be difficult or impossible to achieve. For example, antihistamines are of little benefit in allergic asthma.

The ideal therapy would block initial stimulation of the type 1 reaction, and it is this which hyposensitization attempts to achieve. The idea is not new. Almost 80 years ago, Noon (1911) attempted prophylactic vaccination of patients against allergy by repeated injections of allergen. This attempt followed logically from the successful programmes of disease prophylaxis which had been recently developed by von Behring and Pasteur. Despite the length of experience with this approach, very few drug registrations have been achieved. Ewan *et al.* (1988) comment that: '. . . overall results are poor. Hyposensitisation therapy is unfortunately used indiscriminately and uncritically . . . with many allergen extracts for which there is no proven evidence of benefit . . . controlled studies show convincing evidence for only a limited number of allergens'. A recent issue of the *British National Formulary* (September 1989) comments that the value of hyposensitization is uncertain except for wasp and bee sting allergy, and that administration of allergen extracts is associated with significant risk of anaphylaxis, the risk not being reliably predicted by diagnostic skin testing alone. The CSM has also issued a warning on the use of this therapy, part of which is as follows: 'The CSM has warned that since 1980, in the UK alone, 11 patients, most of whom were young, have died from anaphylaxis caused by allergen extracts and desensitising vaccines; patients with asthma appear to be particularly susceptible . . . Although some vaccines can prevent anaphylactic reactions (e.g. to bee stings) the efficacy of the others is controversial . . .' The warning concludes by advising doctors to balance carefully the risks and potential benefits for each patient and only to carry out this therapy where full cardiopulmonary resuscitation facilities are available. Patients should be observed for at least two hours after injection with allergen, although this stricture has been challenged (Thompson *et al.* 1989).

The classical view of the mechanism of action of hyposensitization therapy, is that injection of allergen stimulates the production of specific IgG antibodies which block the interaction between allergen and IgE. Much recent research has therefore been directed towards reducing the adverse effects of hyposensitization therapy by chemical modification of allergens to reduce their allergenicity (IgE stimulation) and enhance their immunogenicity (IgG stimulation). Another approach has been to administer specific IgG just prior to initiation of hyposensitization therapy in an effort to provide 'blocking antibodies' to prevent systemic IgE-mediated effects whilst the endogenous production of IgG is getting going in response to the hyposensitizing agent. Examples of both types of study are included in the methodological survey below.

In view of the clinical dangers outlined above, as well as the very large number of allergic individuals whose quality of life could be improved by these methods if they were successful, a methodological survey of hyposensitization trials appears justified.

Special features of hyposensitization trials

A number of special features confront the trialist undertaking a clinical study of hyposensitization therapy. These were considered recently by a WHO/IUIS (International Union of Immunological Societies) working group (Thompson *et al.* 1989) which drew particular attention to the following points:

(1) The need for standardized allergen preparations;

(2) The need for better definitions of the desired level of benefit (see question 2 of scoring system);

(3) Variation in the patients' perception of their symptoms and, consequently, the role of objective challenge tests and *in vitro* immunological tests for specific IgE or IgG (see questions 22 and 23);

(4) Differences between the natural and presumed level of exposure to the allergen and the co-existence of other allergies in patients undergoing treatment for a single allergy (see question 27);

(5) The selection of appropriate patients (see question 12) with the following characteristics:
   - an allergy which has been proven to be IgE mediated;
   - allergen avoidance measures have failed;
   - existing drugs have failed or have unacceptable side-effects;
   - limited spectrum of allergen sensitivities;
   - likely to comply with the complex regimen;
   - absence of diseases of the immune system;
   - absence of conditions, such as hypertension, which would make it difficult to handle likely adverse events;
   - absence of concomitant therapies, such as beta-blockers, which would make it difficult to handle adverse events;
   - pregnancy.

(6) The need for a carefully planned dosage regimen, often extending over prolonged periods of time and involving dosage escalation, whilst carefully monitoring for adverse events which may necessitate temporary modification of the regimen in individual patients (see questions 17, 19, 24, 25, and 29). Most patients will show some degree of local reaction which is not regarded as a contra-

indication to further treatment. A significant number of patients show systemic reactions such as asthma, rhinitis and urticaria, hypotension, or angioedema. The WHO/IUIS working party recommended that in such cases, the next dose should be reduced to a third in an effort to avoid life-threatening anaphylactic reactions, although they point out that only 6 of 26 fatalities reported to the CSM had a history of adverse reactions to prior injections. The WHO/IUIS working party also suggested that a dosage reduction was advisable in the case of severe local reactions.

Each of these points, except for the first one which relates to drug design rather than trial design, is considered in the following section under the question indicated.

Outcome of scoring

Fifteen RCTs, involving approximately 600 evaluable patients, were included in this survey. NRCTs were not included in this survey because of the generally accepted need for randomized control trials for testing this sort of therapy. Such studies readily gain ethical acceptance when no existing therapy has proven to be effective for a particular allergen or group of patients.

The scores achieved by the 15 hyposensitization RCTs ranged from 20 to 67 per cent with a mean of 43.67 per cent and a median of 41 per cent. There was no correlation ($R^2 = 0.113$) between score and year of publication, which ranged from 1984 to 1989. Table 8.1 shows which questions most frequently achieved each possible score.

Questions which usually scored '2'

Some of the patient selection criteria (question 12; point 5 on p. 181) from the WHO/IUIS report were usually satisfied (IgE-mediated nature; exclusion of multiple allergy), whilst some were less frequently mentioned (prior treatment failure; exclusion of concomitant conditions; likelihood of compliance). Most of the studies surveyed used skin testing to determine allergen sensitivity, the IgE-mediated nature of the allergy being indicated by the characteristic type I reaction of wheal and flare. Several studies correlated the seasonal appearance of allergens with patient history to confirm the clinical relevance of the skin test findings. For example, in a trial of mould allergy hypo-

Table 8.1 Score frequencies for each question

Question number	Subject of question	Score frequency (per cent) 2	1	0	Sample* number
Questions which usually scored '2'					
3	Informed consent before randomization	86.67	6.67	6.67	15
5	Blindness of patients to treatment	86.67	6.67	6.67	15
6	Blindness of clinicians to treatment	80.00	13.33	6.67	15
12	Reporting of patient selection criteria	60.00	33.33	6.67	15
13	Reporting of patient numbers	73.33	13.33	13.33	15
17	Reporting of dosage regimen	53.33	33.33	13.33	15
22	Objectivity of clinical monitoring	46.67	33.33	20.00	15
23	Relevance of immunological monitoring	66.67	33.33	0.00	12
25	Adverse immunological event reporting	46.67	33.33	20.00	15
27	Baseline comparison of patients	46.67	6.67	46.67	15
28	Reporting of results	60.00	33.33	6.67	15
Questions which usually scored '1':					
2	Definition of endpoints	33.33	53.33	13.33	15
15	Patient withdrawal log	28.57	42.86	28.57	7
18	Identity of comparator in blind studies	28.57	35.71	35.71	14
20	Exclusion of concomitant therapies	26.67	46.67	26.67	15
21	Length of washout in crossover studies	0.00	100.00	0.00	1
30	Dropout accounting	16.67	50.00	33.33	12
Questions which usually scored '0'					
1	Number of endpoints	26.67	20.00	53.33	15
4	Method of randomization	0.00	6.67	93.33	15
7	Blindness to ongoing results	6.67	6.67	86.67	15
8	Choice of statistical methods	13.33	33.33	53.33	15
9	Homogeneity check on multicentre data	0.00	0.00	100.00	4
10	Trial size by power calculation	0.00	0.00	100.00	15
11	Other reason for trial size	0.00	0.00	100.00	15
14	Patient reject log	6.67	13.33	80.00	15
16	Exclusion of concomitant diseases	13.33	20.00	66.67	15
19	Interruptions to drug administration	6.67	33.33	60.00	15
24	Close monitoring for adverse events	13.33	33.33	53.33	15
26	Uniformity of multicentre evaluations	0.00	0.00	100.00	4
29	Adverse event reporting	6.67	33.33	60.00	15
31	Statistical reporting	0.00	46.67	53.33	15
32	Results in terms of trial size	6.67	6.67	86.67	15

*Sample number = the number of trials scored minus the number for which the question was not applicable

sensitization, patients were selected who 'were either symptom-free (the majority) or had only minimal asthma outside the Cladosporium season' (Malling *et al*. 1986). Some trials included specific IgE determinations to confirm the nature of the type I reaction.

The same methods can be used to eliminate patients with multiple allergies. Ortolani *et al*. (1984) gave one of the fullest descriptions of patient selection criteria: '(1) Positive SPT and RAST for grass pollens and clinical correspondence of symptoms with the seasonal pollenation pattern; (2) negative SPT and RAST for Bermuda grass pollen and for all other inhalent allergens (pollens, mites, moulds etc); (3) presence of bronchial asthma and rhinitis; (4) no previous specific immunotherapy; (5) no other chronic disease; (6) no pregnancy in progress; (7) residence and work in the Milan district where the pollen count was determined.' (NB: SPT = skin prick test; RAST = radioallergosorbent test). One study (Marks *et al*. 1987) attempted hyposensitization for a type IV allergy to poison ivy. Patients were selected according to history and delayed-type skin test.

As explained on p. 181, trials of hyposensitization therapy often involve careful tailoring of a complex dosage regimen according to the individual patient's response. Most of the trials surveyed included details of the planned regimen (question 17), although rather fewer presented details of the interruptions due to side-effects or other reasons (question 19; point 6 on p. 181). Whilst most studies reported the initial and final doses of allergen in the planned regimen, several did not include the size of the dosage increments used between these limits. Ohman *et al*. (1984) gave a clear account of a typical hyposensitization regimen using 1/10 and 1/100 dilutions of a cat allergen preparation (13 units of allergen per ml): 'an initial subcutaneous injection of 0.05 cc of 1/100 dilution was administered and at weekly intervals the dose was doubled until the maximum tolerated dose was achieved or 0.3 cc of the undiluted preparation was administered'. Some reports included a table summarizing the regimen (e.g. Grammer *et al*. 1987). (Several reports did not include the route of administration, referring only to 'injections'. This point was not scored, however, due to the universal use of the subcutaneous route). The surveyed studies included examples of RUSH (Bousquet *et al*. 1987*a*) and CLUSTER (Malling *et al*. 1986) regimens.

The methods available for clinical monitoring (question 22; point 3 on p. 181) include the subjective reporting of symptoms by patients, the quantity of symptomatic medication used by the patients and the recording of more objective variables such as nasal airway resistance or forced expiratory volume. Monitoring may be performed during either natural exposure or experimental challenge with the allergen. Nasal, bronchial, skin and conjunctival provocation tests are all routinely used, although it has been suggested that some of these tests may not be truly quantitative (Moller *et al.* 1984).

In several of the studies surveyed, efforts were made to enhance the objectivity of the data. For example, Corrado *et al.* (1989) substantiated the individual patient records of their use of symptomatic medication by counting the remaining tablets or weighing nasal spray canisters. Some trialists performed studies of the reproducibility of the provocation test methods they employed. Bertelsen *et al.* (1989) checked the comparability of bronchial provocation test results obtained two weeks apart in a separate study on nine patients, whilst the conjunctival provocation test used by Moller *et al.* (1986) was extensively investigated in a prior publication (Moller *et al.* 1984). In the latter study, the information obtained on the scatter of observations made it possible to generate graphs showing the number of patients required to detect a range of differences in allergen sensitivities between two treatment groups. These statistical power calculations will assist with the design of future trials. Muller *et al.* (1987) referred to training patients to perform the PEFR (Peak Expiratory Flow Rate) manoeuvre until repeatable results were obtained. In the same study visual analogue scales were used on two occasions to assess patients' symptoms over the preceding 2 weeks. The trialists state that on the second occasion, the patient was not able to see his first test. This reduces the likelihood of a biased record. The majority of the studies included monitoring of allergen-specific IgE and IgG (question 23; point 3 on p. 181). The most popular theory for the mechanism of hyposensitization regards the IgG as 'blocking antibodies'.

The major concern about hyposensitization therapy is the incidence of adverse immunological events (question 25; point 6 on p. 181). Most reports therefore included information about local reactions (wheal, flare, erythema, etc.), and systemic effects such as urticaria, angioedema, asthma, and anaphylaxis. Ewan *et al.* (1988), for example, included a detailed account of the incidence of each type of reaction (8 anaphylactic, 23 other generalized, and 20 local reactions in a sample of 205 injections), the treatments applied (adrenalin, oxygen, nebulized salbutamol, intramuscular hydrocortisone) and the outcome (even the most severe reaction had almost completely subsided within 20 minutes). The search for and reporting of other types of adverse event was less well carried-out and is discussed on p. 191.

Question 27 relates to the reporting of baseline comparability of the treatment groups. Baseline data such as age, sex, IgE titre (RAST), provocation test outcome, and history (severity, duration) of rhinitis or asthma were generally clearly reported for the studies surveyed (e.g. Bousquet *et al.* 1987*a*). Some reports, however, merely stated that there was no statistically significant difference between the treatment groups on such criteria, but gave neither the data nor the test used nor the *p*-value. This scored '0'.

For some trials the principal endpoint involved a provocation test. Others, however, involved monitoring patients symptoms in response to natural exposure. In such studies it is important to establish that the level of exposure to allergen of the patients in the treatment groups is comparable. This can be assumed, for example, for a trial of pollen hyposensitization, when the trial is conducted in a single centre over one pollen season. Studies of allergy to house dust or cat dander, however, may involve patients whose domestic exposure covers a wide range. Exposure to allergen may change during the timecourse of the trial. It is therefore advisable to estimate exposure in samples of household dust on two or three occasions during the course of the trial. Bertelsen *et al.* (1989) measured the levels of dog and cat allergen in domestic dust samples before and after 9 months of immunotherapy. They found little change in most of the 27 participants' homes but three in the active and one in the control group were exposed to increased levels after 9 months, whilst one of the active group patients had practically eliminated animal dander allergen from his home. Trials of hyposensitization to such antigens which did not include any comment about exposure scored '0' regardless of any other baseline data presented. Hence, as many trials scored '0' as '2' for question 27.

The results were usually clearly reported (question 28) with the proviso discussed on p. 192 that it would be helpful to have more information about the outcome per patient in relation to the dosage regimen actually received after the various interruptions and modifications dictated by the patients' reactions to therapy. The range of cumulative doses received by the patients in a single trial can cover an enormous range, for example 5695 to 73 800 units (Bousquet *et al.* 1987*b*). The primary endpoint of the trial would remain the determination of whether or not a particular planned regimen, administered as far as adverse events allow, improves the condition of the group of participants. Information about outcome in relation to dose would provide useful additional information which could be of value in planning further experiments or trials.

As with the other therapeutic areas, the number of patients enrolled and evaluated was usually reported clearly (question 13), although a flow-chart might have aided comprehensibility in one or two trials with complicated designs.

Virtually all trials were conducted double-blind (questions 3, 5, and 6) which is essential for removing bias from subjective evaluation of symptoms. The related issue of placebo identity (question 18) scored rather less well and is discussed on p. 188; questions 4 and 7 (dealing with the randomization method and code-breaking, respectively) are covered on p. 190. The scope for very large placebo effects was illustrated by Corrado *et al.* (1989) in which the percentage of symptom-free patient days doubled between baseline and 5 months (according to patients' morning diaries) in the control group.

Questions which usually scored '1'

For the majority of the studies surveyed, it was clear what variables were being monitored and, where appropriate, scoring systems for symptoms and/or medication were defined by the trialists (e.g. Price *et al.* 1984). Endpoints were less clear in terms of a desired level of benefit (question 2; point 2 on p. 181) such as the criteria for defining a patient as 'significantly improved' or regarding a result as 'clinically significant'. This is especially important when laboratory challenge tests are used as the endpoint rather than natural exposure. For example, a study of dog and cat allergens (Bertelsen *et al.* 1989) involved the use of bronchial provocation testing (BPT) to assess response to hyposensitization therapy. The trialists state that the aim of the study was 'to establish whether (hyposensitization) therapy can be recommended as a supplement to conventional medical therapy'. At 9 months, 'an average patient' tolerated five times as much allergen in the BPT as they had done prior to treatment. Whilst this result is statistically significant should it be regarded as clinically significant? Is it a sufficient increase to carry typical patients above a typical level of exposure? Challenge tests are very useful in terms of convenience and standardization, but there needs to be a way of relating the outcome to everyday experience. One way of doing this which carries the implication of clinical significance is to monitor the usage of symptomatic treatments during the trial period (e.g. Price *et al.* 1984).

Clearly, there is a marked difference between trials of, for example, anti-cancer agents and hyposensitization therapy in terms of endpoints. In the former, a small improvement in life expectancy and quality is worth knowing about, whereas in the latter, quite large improvements in experimental tolerance may be worthless if the patient is still sensitive at the level of environmental exposure. This needs to be reflected in the endpoint definitions. For example, 'a patient will be regarded as a treatment success if their provocation test result improves by at least

x-fold (outside the allergen season) *and* their use of symptomatic treatments (specify) decreases y-fold using a specified scoring system (inside
the season)'. In this way, one source of controversy about hyposensitization therapy, whereby those who review the results of provocation
testing would conclude that it is more successful than those who considered the overall impact in clinical practice, would be removed. In
addition, the requirement for a similar trend in two quite different
endpoints in order for a patient to be classified as a success would add
credibility to the results. The use of endpoints which encompass several
observations would also have the advantage of reducing the number of
statistical tests (see discussion of question 1 below).

Scadding and Brostoff (1986) utilized a crossover design and simply
asked the patients which treatment they considered best alleviated their
symptoms. The results of objective assessments were then correlated.
So long as such studies are conducted blind and appropriate considera-
tion is given to possible carry-over of effect from one treatment phase
to the other, then this endpoint does carry clinical significance. Ohman
et al. (1984), in a study of cat-induced asthma, placed treated patients
in a room with live cats and used a scale for subjective assessment
which had clear clinical relevance: 0—no symptoms; 1—trivial or barely
noticeable; 2—definitely present but not bothersome; 3—bothersome
but not disabling or intolerable; 4—disabling and/or intolerable. Such
studies must be conducted strictly blind and there is the possibility of,
for example, panic attacks complicating the results.

Questions 15 (withdrawal log) and 30 (lost to follow-up analysis)
scored '1' most frequently for the same range of reasons observed for
the other therapeutic areas such as: not indicating the reasons for
withdrawal by treatment group; not indicating whether or not all of the
patients who were contributing data at the start of a timecourse were
still doing so at the end (i.e. censorship); simply stating that a number
of patients were lost to follow-up without indicating at what stage of the
regimen they were lost or the outcome of treatment at that point.
Perhaps the clearest stated policy for dealing with patients lost to
follow-up was given by Corrado *et al.* (1989): 'Because many withdrawals in one treatment group may improve results in that group as
treatment failures leave, allowance was made for withdrawals in the
analysis of the data. A conservative method was used, substituting a
patient's last available observation at all subsequent time points, thus
ensuring no bias in favour of the active therapy.'

Blindness requires identity of the various treatments, which in many
cases included a placebo. The majority of the studies reported the
nature of the placebo but rather few noted whether or not it was

identical in appearance to the active treatment (question 18). This question scored '2', '1' or '0' with roughly equal frequency (see Table 8.1). Several studies used placebos containing histamine to mimic the reactions some patients show to hyposensitization therapy (Corrado *et al.* 1989; Ewan *et al.* 1988; Bousquet *et al.* 1987a; Grammer *et al.* 1987; Ohman *et al.* 1984 and Malling *et al.* 1986). Some (e.g. Ewan *et al.* 1988) administered a range of concentrations of histamine to mimic the escalating dosage of allergen, whilst others mentioned the use of riboflavin (Ortolani *et al.* 1984) or caramelization (Malling *et al.* 1986), although they do not say that the final preparation was identical to the active treatment. Grammer *et al.* (1987) used caramelized glucose and histamine which was 'visually indistinguishable'. Muller *et al.* (1987) used chemically modified and un-modified honeybee venom preparations which were 'visually identical' in both the lyophilized and reconstituted state.

Most trials mentioned the exclusion of concomitant therapies (question 20). Some trials excluded all other medication (Scadding and Brostoff 1986) or limited the range of concomitant medication to a small number of nasal sprays and antihistamines (Ewan *et al.* 1988). Several excluded those who had received prior specific immunotherapy (e.g. Ortolani *et al.* 1984). Given that the mechanism of hyposensitization has not been firmly established, it would be advisable to exclude patients who are receiving any other immunomodulators, whether stimulatory or suppressive.

There was only one crossover trial amongst the 15 RCTs surveyed (Scadding and Brostoff 1986) involving 2 weeks on one treatment (active or placebo) followed by a 2-week washout period (question 21) before 2 weeks on the other treatment. The trialists stated that 'the effect of this form of therapy appears quickly (2–4 days) and wears off over a week after stopping', although no data was shown or reference given to support this statement. [Price *et al.* (1984) randomized patients to placebo or active treatments for 1 year and then re-randomized those who had been in the active group to a further period of placebo or active treatment. This constituted a trial of treatment withdrawal at 1 year rather than a crossover study. Meanwhile, the patients who had received placebo in the first year were given active treatment in year 2.]

Questions which usually scored '0'

The majority of the studies had more than two endpoints (question 1), such as the outcome of provocation testing, symptom self-assessment and medication usage. The use of combined endpoints as discussed on

p. 188 would circumvent this problem. The other way around this difficulty is to state which endpoint is the primary one (e.g. Price *et al.* 1984—requirement for symptomatic medication).

None of the studies clearly indicated the method of randomization used (question 4) and few gave an indication that the code was not broken until the end of the trial (question 7).

All of the questions relating to statistics usually scored '0' (questions 8, 10, 11, 31, and 32). The reporting of statistical analyses suffered from the usual range of criticisms mentioned for the other therapeutic areas such as: quoting attainment of threshold p-values rather than the actual p-value; not indicating whether a scatter range represents standard error or standard deviation; not calculating confidence intervals where appropriate. Trial size was virtually never considered. Marks *et al.* (1987) included a *post-hoc* power calculation, having failed to see a statistically significant incidence of hyposensitization with 84 patients.

For two trials (Muller *et al.* 1987 and Bousquet *et al.* 1987*c*), the primary endpoint was not the demonstration of improved efficacy for the new treatment but, instead, the demonstration of improved safety (i.e. fewer systemic reactions during administration) with at least equivalent efficacy for the new treatment. A method for calculating the number of patients required to set statistical limits upon the equivalence of two treatments was given by Pocock (1983). Large numbers of patients are usually required, certainly far greater than the numbers used in Muller *et al.* (1987) and Bousquet *et al.* (1987*c*). It follows that there is a marked probability of the observed equivalence of the treatments being due to chance and that there is really a difference in efficacy between them. Consider, for example, the design of a new trial to confirm the results obtained by Muller *et al.* (1987) in which a challenge with a live honeybee was used to test efficacy. The frequency of systemic response to this challenge can be assumed to be 2 out of 14 on the older treatment based on the results of Muller *et al.* (1987). Thus 85.7 per cent of participants who receive the older treatment will *not* suffer a systemic reaction. Let us suppose that we wish to prove, with 95 per cent probability, that the new treatment is no more than 10 per cent inferior to the older treatment in this respect. According to the method of Pocock (1983), 194 patients per treatment group would be necessary and even then, there would be a 20 per cent risk of the new treatment appearing to be more than 10 per cent inferior even if it was really the same. Far larger numbers would be required to reduce this risk.

Only four of the fifteen studies surveyed were multicentre trials. None of them referred to either the homogeneity of the data by centre (question 9) or to measures to ensure the standardization of evaluations (question 26).

Almost none of the studies included any form of reject log (question 14). Malling *et al.* (1986) reported that their patient population was selected from 62 adults whose history suggested mould allergy (exacerbation of asthma during the Cladosporium season). 25 showed a positive bronchial provocation test, of whom 23 gave informed consent. Ortolani *et al.* (1984) stated that, of 200 potential participants, only 15 fitted the list of seven selection criteria. The latter trial therefore tested the hyposensitization therapy on a very small and specialized sample of the patient population. When considering the possible generalizability of the results it would be helpful to know the frequency with which the seven selection criteria were violated. However impressive the results, further work will be required to establish safety and efficacy in the general population.

Three questions relating to adverse events (16, 24, and 29; point 6 on p. 181) most frequently scored '0' in this sample of 15 RCTs. Whilst some studies excluded patients with one or two specified concomitant diseases which might be expected to have a direct bearing upon efficacy or safety of trial therapy, few mentioned the general state of health of the patients (question 16). Exceptions included Grammer *et al.* (1987), where patients with allergic rhinitis who were otherwise healthy were selected on the basis of: history, physical examination, ESR, complete and differential blood count, and liver and renal biochemistry. Few studies reported looking for adverse events (question 24) other than the immunological events discussed in question 25 above. Grammer *et al.* (1987) repeated the above battery of laboratory tests after the final injection, and a similar range of tests were also used in Moller *et al.* (1986) and Marks *et al.* (1987). Prior to each injection, Corrado *et al.* (1989) asked each patient: 'Did you notice anything unusual after the last injection?'. Few studies mentioned whether or not any adverse events were seen (question 29) other than the immunological events. Minor gastro-intestinal disturbances (nausea, colic or diarrhoea) were observed with an oral pollen preparation (Moller *et al.* 1986) whilst there were isolated reports of headaches (Price *et al.* 1984 and Malling *et al.* 1986), weakness (Price *et al.* 1984), and depression (Malling *et al.* 1986). The three studies which monitored blood chemistry reported no changes (Grammer *et al.* 1987 and Marks *et al.* 1987) or occasional values outside the normal range but no difference between active and control groups (Moller *et al.* 1986).

Most studies mentioned the need for dosage modification due to unwanted immune effects, but few gave either specific criteria for

dosage interruption or modification in the 'Methods' section or details of
the dosage regimen actually recieved by patients in the 'Results' section
(question 19; point 6 on p. 181). Whether or not there were interruptions
for reasons other than adverse events was generally not mentioned.

Ewan *et al.* (1988) set out their criteria for dosage modification as
follows: 'the regime was modified if there was a history of recent
respiratory infection or worsening of asthma (dose usually omitted and
the same dose given next visit) or any intercurrent illness (dose halved
or omitted). The dose was reduced if the peak flow had fallen more
than 10 per cent below the patient's baseline, even in the absence of
clinical change. The dose was reduced if a generalized allergic reaction
had occurred to the previous injection (the reduction depending upon
the type and severity of the reaction) or the same dose was repeated if a
large local reaction had occurred'.

Given that the dosage regimen received by each participant in a trial
of hyposensitization therapy is individually tailored, according to the
reaction of their immune system to the allergen, it would be helpful
when comparing the outcome of several trials to know what dosage
regimens were actually received by the participants in each. Several
trials reported the range of cumulative doses received and these can
cover an enormous range, for example 5695 to 73 800 units (Bousquet
et al. 1987*b*) or 2900 to 13 500 units (Bousquet *et al.* 1987*a*). Some
studies reported the dose received and the outcome of clinical endpoints for each patient (e.g. Bertelsen *et al.* 1989 and Bousquet *et al.*
1987*b*) in the form of simple charts showing symptom score or provocation test outcome against dose received. [Bertelsen *et al.* (1989) observed
a correlation between maintenance dose at 9 months and provocation
test outcome, whilst Bousquet *et al.* (1987*b*) saw no correlation between
total dose and symptom scores or provocation test outcome.] Other
reports included only summarized information such as: 'Five patients
receiving polymerised ragweed had a total of seven large local reactions
that required dosage modification. These patients required a total of five
additional injections' (Grammer *et al.* 1987). It would be interesting to
know more about the modifications to the regimen and the outcome in
these patients. There appears to be plenty of scope for improving the
reporting of the dosage regimens actually received and thus facilitating
the comparison of trials.

QC

Three of the questions relating to quality control of data were applied
to these reports. None of the 15 RCT reports mentioned data auditing

(question (i)). Neither of the multicentre trials in which laboratory determinations were made mentioned whether or not samples were sent to a central laboratory, and so question (iv) (effects of the transportation of samples upon the result) was 'NA' in both cases. One trial report (Ohman *et al.* 1984) mentions testing patients for blindness (question (ii)). Each patient was asked to fill out a form that indicated whether they believed they had received the active or placebo treatment.

Mechanism of action

This has been reviewed by de Weck (1985) and is discussed in the WHO-IUIS report (Thompson *et al.* 1989). The classical view is that injection of allergen stimulates the production of specific IgG antibodies which block the interaction between allergen and IgE. The most compelling evidence for this mechanism comes from studies such as Bousquet *et al.* (1987*c*) (see above) in which administration of IgG from beekeepers could prevent the systemic adverse events associated with honeybee venom injections. Whilst it is easy to envisage how IgG and IgE could compete for allergen in the blood and hence prevent systemic events, de Weck has questioned the ability of IgG to interfere with events in the skin or mucosa. Perhaps IgA could be involved. Interestingly, beekeeper IgG failed to reduce the incidence of large local reactions in response to honeybee venom (Bousquet *et al.* 1987*c*). Nor is a correlation between serum IgG and clinical benefit routinely observed in all patients. Turner *et al.* (1984) investigated the levels of IgG, IgE, and IgA in children undergoing hyposensitization therapy for house dust mite allergy (Price *et al.* 1984—see above). There was a slight rise in mean IgG titre amongst the patients receiving hyposensitization therapy and a slight fall amongst the placebo patients, but there was no correlation between the magnitude of this effect and the patients' asthma. Nor was any consistent effect upon either IgE or IgA levels observed.

The production of IgE follows from a complex interaction of antigen-presenting cells, helper and suppressor T cells and B cells. IgE is presumably also linked into the idiotype-anti-idiotype network. Various suggestions for down regulation of IgE synthesis involving these mechanisms have been made, although these are confounded by the frequent lack of correlation between IgE titre and clinical benefit in individual cases. Inhibition of inflammatory effector cells (mast cells, basophils, etc.) has also been suggested.

Appendix 8.1 List of hyposensitization trials included in this survey

Test drug	Test patients evaluated	Control treatment	Control patients evaluated	Outcome of scoring	Reference
ONE POLLEN EX	14	PBO	16	GA	Moller et al. (1986)
MIXED POLLEN EX	8	PBO	7	GA	Ortolani et al. (1984)
MIXED POLLEN EX	19 ⎫	PBO=HIST	11	GA	Bousquet et al. (1987a)
ONE POLLEN EX	15 ⎭				
GLUT-POLLEN EX	?	PBO=HIST	?	GA	Grammer et al. (1987)
FORM-POLLEN EX	?	PBO	?	LS	Bousquet et al. (1987b)
HDM EX	?	PBO=HIST	?	GA	Ewan et al. (1988)
HDM EX	X18	PBO	X18	GA	Scadding and Brostoff (1986)
ALG-HDM EX	22	PBO=ALG+/−HIST*	29	GA	Corrado et al. (1989)
TYR, GLUT-HDM	27	PBO=TYR	24	GA	Price et al. (1984)
DOG & CAT EX	14	NONE	13	GA	Bertelsen et al. (1989)
CAT PELT EX	9	PBO=HIST	8	GA	Ohman et al. (1984)
BKgG + HBV	20	HBV	7	GA	Bousquet et al. (1987c)
mPEG-HBV	17	HBV	14	GA	Muller et al. (1987)
CLADOSPORIUM EX	11	PBO=HIST	11	HS	Malling et al. (1986)
PDC + HDC	42	PBO	42	GA	Marks et al. (1987)

Key

Allergens:

HBV = honey bee venom
HDM = house dust mite
PDC+HDC = Pentadecylcatechol and heptadecylcatechol (PDC is the allergen in Poison Ivy resin)

Allergen derivatization:

ALG = Alginate
FORM = Formalin
GLUT = Glutaraldehyde
mPEG = Monomethoxy polyethylene glycol
TYR = Tyrosine

Other:

BKgG = Beekeepers' gamma globulin
EX = Extract
HIST = Histamine
PBO = Placebo
X = Crossover trial
* = Histamine added to some placebo vials at random

9

Conclusions and recommendations

The 190 trials surveyed in this book represent the accumulated clinical experience of immunological agents gained from 147 167 evaluable patients between 1980 and 1989. During this time, the remarkable range of ingenious ways dreamed up to influence the immune system prove human creativity is alive and well and living in clinical immunology! Some of the more impressive approaches include the *ex vivo* stimulation of killer cells (Rosenberg *et al.* 1987), the use of aggressive chemotherapy while a sample of bone marrow has been temporarily removed from the body, and the use of colony stimulating factors to speed its re-establishment (Brandt *et al.* 1988) and the exquisite specificity of anti-idiotypes (Meeker *et al.* 1985). Meanwhile, hyposensitization therapy continues to be a puzzle within an enigma.

It is hoped this survey of clinical trial technique will help to ensure immunological agents are tested in the kind of quality trials they deserve. It would be a great shame if an ingenious method were discarded because a poorly designed trial failed to demonstrate efficacy. Equally, it should be remembered that the immune system, even in the healthy state, is not yet fully understood and the possibility of profound side-effects occurring when tinkering with the diseased system demands scrupulous reporting of adverse events. The complexity of the immune system and the constellation of effects induced by most immunological agents mean that clinical trial technique must be rigorous. The experimental system is quite complex enough without poor methodology clouding the picture. Perhaps differences in technique could be responsible for some of the observed variation in the results obtained with, for example, interferon in hairy cell leukaemia (Chapter 5) or hyposensitization therapy (Chapter 8).

Lessons learned

The outcome of this survey suggests the principal means by which clinical trials of immunological agents can be improved are as follows.

More attention should be paid to the avoidance of bias

Trial size must be determined at the outset to avoid the bias introduced by stopping the trial when the results look encouraging rather than when a predetermined enrolment has been attained. For RCTs, size should preferably be determined by means of a power calculation in order to avoid type II error (i.e. concluding there is no difference between treatments when one exists). It is remarkable how few trials used these methods. Surely those funding the trials, usually the manufacturers, would like to know (and minimize) the probability of an expensive trial failing to demonstrate efficacy for a product which does in fact work! There are, of course, several other legitimate factors which may limit the size of a trial, including rarity of the disease or the number of cases becoming ill in an epidemic. On the other hand, limiting trial size in an attempt to avoid the expense of a large trial is a false economy.

Once trial size has been determined, the study must be left to run its course to completion. Early publication, for example, before some of the patients have finished 5 years follow-up in a cancer trial, is not acceptable as discussed in Chapter 5. If it is essential to obtain a result as quickly as possible, then sequential statistical methods are available, in which each new event is added to an ongoing analysis, in such a way as to avoid the risks usually associated with repeated analyses (Whitehead 1983).

The opportunity for bias can be further decreased by reducing the number of endpoints and stating at the outset which endpoint should be regarded as the primary outcome. Otherwise there is scope for choosing *post-hoc* the most favourable of several endpoints and promoting it as the primary result. Trial size should be calculated based upon the projected incidence of the primary endpoint. Endpoint definitions should always be given, including the methods to be used to monitor them, criteria for establishing the cause of death (where appropriate) and the level of efficacy which would be regarded as *clinically* significant, as opposed to *statistically* significant. Well defined endpoints avoid debate about outcome from which biased decisions may arise.

Finally, the scope for bias can be further reduced in non-blind RCTs by gaining informed consent without knowledge of randomization allocation. This was virtually never mentioned. If the patients are aware of allocation then it is possible to envisage circumstances in which the treatment groups would accrue quite different populations as discussed in Chapter 4.

Statistical technique should be improved

This can best be achieved by keeping the design of the trial as simple as possible in order to avoid the need for sophisticated statistical methodology. Whenever possible, there should be no more than two treatment groups and one principal endpoint.

Involve a statistician from the outset to help to design the trial and ensure that all those involved in planning and funding the trial are aware of the implications of the statistician's input. For example, if provision is made for periodic interim analyses, a stricter level of significance than $p = 0.05$ is required for a result to be regarded as significant. It is prudent to ensure everyone understands this at the outset. Trying to explain to the managing director, at the *end* of an expensive trial, that a result yielding $p = 0.05$ cannot be accepted after all, because this was the outcome of the third interim analysis, is not recommended!

Report confidence intervals whenever possible, always give exact *p*-values, and indicate whether a scatter range is the standard deviation or the standard error.

Avoid historical controls

There was an example in Chapter 5 of a trial in which the result obtained from comparison with a randomized control group was quite different from the result which would have been obtained with a historical control group (Lessner *et al.* 1984). The control group performed far better than expected according to historical data. Thus, no advantage was observed for the active treatment in the randomized study, but a comparison with historical controls would have indicated a benefit for the active treatment.

Improve adverse event reporting

In particular, pay more attention to adverse immunological events as discussed above and in Chapter 4. Report the question used to elicit subjective events because the frequency with which some events are reported may depend upon how the patient is asked about them. Avoid dismissing the adverse events observed in interferon trials as being 'the same as usually observed'. This engenders a lazy attitude which could mean that low-frequency events are overlooked or not reported.

*Provide more information about rejected patients and
censorship*

Provide more information on how the chosen population relates to the
general population with the disease by providing a patient reject log.
This will facilitate an understanding of the applicability of the results.
Indicate more clearly the numbers of patients lost to follow-up and the
reasons. Remember that patients may drop-out because of lack of
efficacy, thus influencing the final result. Analysis of the efficacy is
incomplete without an analysis of drop-outs.

Employ quality control methods

Checks on patients' compliance with the dosage regimen, to check that
the trial medication is being given a fair appraisal, need to be performed and reported far more frequently. In Chapter 5, a study was
reported in which cancer patients were asked to take a 600 mg dose of
aspirin four times a day whilst receiving interferon from the trialists
(Creagan *et al*. 1988). Less than half (41 per cent) of the patients took
at least 90 per cent of the aspirin regimen, the usual reason for non-
compliance being nausea. This illustrates the level of compliance which
can be expected, even with highly motivated cancer patients taking an
orally administered drug. How much more non-compliance might be
observed with, for example, self-administered injections, less severe
illnesses (i.e. less motivation) or side-effects such as depression and
lethargy.

Multicentre studies would benefit from methods to standardize
evaluations between the centres. These were rarely reported, yet the
greater the variation in the data the more difficult it is to discern a
treatment benefit. This can be thought of as a reduction in the 'signal to
noise' ratio of the data and effectively reduces the power of the trial.
The use of a central laboratory in such studies, whilst standardizing
assessments, introduces a further source of variation in the form of the
effects of sample transportation (e.g. 24 hours in a postal sorting office,
perhaps near a heater). Checks for the effects of transportation were
virtually never reported.

Data auditing, to check for unintentional errors, was only explicitly
mentioned in one of the 190 trials included in this survey. If such
methods are employed, in order for the data to be accepted by the US-
FDA, then the trialists may as well mention it in the publication
because it adds a further level of credibility to the results.

Raison d'etre

In conclusion, it is hoped that this book will assist trialists in three ways. Firstly, and most important, it will assist with the design of future trials by drawing lessons from past studies. Secondly, it will help to encourage critical reading of trial literature. Thirdly, by providing, in the form of appendices to each chapter, a catalogue of 190 recent trials it will help the clinician who is new to the area to find quickly a way into the literature.

As explained in Chapter 4, the scoring system was really no more than a checklist of the kind of questions that should be asked when reading clinical trial papers with a critical eye and it was not based upon any absolute indicators of quality. It should therefore be regarded principally as a means of highlighting deficiencies rather than providing an accurate credibility rating for each trial. It is intended that this survey should stimulate constructive discussion of clinical trial methodology rather than debates about the scores achieved by particular studies. A cleaner experimental system will increase the resolution of our observations of immunointervention during the 1990s and hopefully provide us with a set of powerful therapeutic tools with which to enter the next millenium.

References

ABPI (1988). *Guidelines on good clinical research practice.* Association of the British Pharmaceutical Industry, 12 Whitehall, London SW1A 2DY, England.

Adams, C. P., Cohen, E. J., Albrecht, J., and Laibson, P. R. (1984). Interferon treatment of adenoviral conjunctivitis. *American Journal of Ophthalmology*, **98**, 429–32.

Ahn, Y. S., Harrington, W. J., Simon, S., Mylvaganam, R., Pall, L. M., and So, A. G. (1983). Danazol for the treatment of idiopathic thrombocytopaenia purpura. *New England Journal of Medicine*, **308**, 1396–9.

Ahre, A., Bjorkholm, M., Mellstedt, H., Brenning, G., Engstedt, L., Gahrton, G. *et al.* (1984). Human leukocyte interferon and intermittent high-dose melphalan-prednisone administration in the treatment of multiple myeloma: a randomised clinical trial from the Myeloma Group of Central Sweden. *Cancer Treatment Reports*, **68**, 1331–8.

American Rheumatism Association (1965). The co-operating clinics committee of the American Rheumatism Association, a seven day variability study of 499 patients with peripheral Rheumatoid Arthritis. *Arthritis and Rheumatism*, **8**, 302–34.

Amor, B., Dougados, M., Mery, C., Dardenne, M., and Bach, J. F. (1987). Nonathymulin in rheumatoid arthritis: two double-blind, placebo controlled trials. *Annals of the Rheumatic Diseases*, **46**, 549–54.

Anon (1990). Largest trials of AIDS drug start in Britain. *New Scientist*, **26th May**, p. 21.

Antman, K. S., Griffin, J. D., Elias, A., Socinski, M. A., Ryan, L., Cannistra, S. A. *et al.* (1988). Effect of recombinant human granulocyte-macrophage colony stimulating factor on chemotherapy-induced myelosuppression. *New England Journal of Medicine*, **319**, 593–8.

Antunes, C. M. F., Mayrink, W., Magalhaes, P. A., Costa, C. A., Melo, M. N., Dias, M. *et al.* (1986). Controlled field trials of a vaccine against New World cutaneous leishmaniasis. *International Journal of Epidemiology*, **15**, 572–80.

Arvin, A. M., Kushner, J. H., Feldman, S., Baehner, R. L., Hammond, D., and Merigan, T. C. (1982). Human leukocyte interferon for the treatment of varicella in children with cancer. *New England Journal of Medicine*, **306**, 761–5.

Assan, R., Feutren, G., Debray-Sachs, M., Quiniou-Debrie, M. C., Laborie, C., Thomas, G. *et al.* (1985). Metabolic and immunological effects of cyclosporin in recently diagnosed type 1 diabetes mellitus. *Lancet*, **i**, 67–71.

Atkins, H. (1966). Address to the Hastings centenary meeting of the BMA. *British Medical Journal*, **2**, 377–9.

Ausobsky, J. R., Evans, M., and Pollock, A. V. (1982). Levamisole and post-operative complications: a controlled clinical trial. *British Journal of Surgery*, **69**, 447–8.

Balkwill, F. (1988). *Cytokines in cancer therapy*. Oxford University Press, Oxford.

BBC (1990) British Broadcasting Corporation, 'Horizon' television science programme, 25th June.

Beasley, R. P., Hwang, L-Y., Lee, G. C-Y., Lan, C-C., Roan, C-H., Huang, F-Y. *et al.* (1983). Prevention of perinatally transmitted hepatitis B virus infections with hepatitis B immune globulin and hepatitis B vaccine. *Lancet*, **ii**, 1099–102.

BenEzra, D., Cohen, E., Chajek, T., Friedman, G., Pizanti, S., de Courten, C. *et al.* (1988). Evaluation of conventional therapy versus cyclosporine A in Behcet's syndrome. *Transplantation Proceedings* XX (3 supplement 4), 136–43.

Ben Yehuda, O., Tomer, Y., and Shoenfeld, Y. (1988). Advances in therapy of autoimmune diseases. *Seminars in Arthritis and Rheumatism*, **17**, 206–20.

Berek, J. S., Hacker, N. F., Lichtenstein, A., Jung, T., Spina, C., Knox, R. M. *et al.* (1985). Intraperitoneal recombinant alpha-interferon for 'salvage' immunotherapy in stage III epithelial ovarian cancer: a Gynecologic Oncology Group Study. *Cancer Research*, **45**, 4447–53.

Bernengo, M. G., Fra, P., Lisa, F., Meregalli, M., and Zina, G. (1983). Thymostimulin therapy in melanoma patients: correlation of immunologic effects and clinical course. *Cancer Immunology and Immunopathology*, **28**, 311–24.

Bertelsen, A., Andersen, J. B., Christensen, J., Ingemann, L., Kristensen, T., and Ostergaard, P. A. A. (1989). Immunotherapy with dog and cat extracts in children. *Allergy*, **44**, 330–5.

Beverley, P. C. L. (1983). Malignant disease. In *Immunology in medicine*, 2nd edn (ed. E. J. Holborrow and W. G. Reeves) pp. 559–74. Academic Press, New York.

Bodey, G. P., Freireich, E. J., McCredie, K. B., Smith, T. L., Gehan, E. A., Gutterman, J. U. *et al.* (1981). Prolonged remissions in adults with acute leukaemia following late intensification chemotherapy and immunotherapy. *Cancer*, **47**, 1937–45.

Bousquet, J., Hejjaoui, A., Skassa-Brociek, W., Guerin, B., Maasch, H. J., Dhivert, H. *et al.* (1987a). Double-blind placebo-controlled immuno-therapy with mixed grass-pollen allergoids. *Journal of Allergy and Clinical Immunology*, **80**, 591–8.

Bousquet, J., Frank, E., Soussana, M., Hejjaoui, A., Maasch, H. J., and Michel, F-B. (1987b). Double-blind placebo-controlled immunotherapy with a high-molecular weight, formalinised allergoid in grass-pollen allergy. *International Archives of Allergy and Applied Immunology*, **82**, 550–2.

Bousquet, J., Fontez, A., Aznar, R., Robinet-Levy, M., and Michel, F-B. (1987c). Combination of passive and active immunisation in honeybee venom immunotherapy. *Journal of Allergy and Clinical Immunology*, **79**, 947–54.

Brandt, S. J., Peters, W. P., Atwater, S. K., Kurtzberg, J., Borowitz, M. J., Jones, R. B. *et al.* (1988). Effect of recombinant human granulocyte-macrophage colony stimulating factor on haematopoietic reconstitution after high-dose chemotherapy and autologous bone-marrow transplantation. *New England Journal of Medicine*, **318**, 869–76.

Breslow, N. (1970). A generalised Kruskal–Wallis test for comparing K samples subject to unequal patterns of censorship. *Biometrika*, **57**, 579–94.

Buelli, M., Cortelazzo, S., Viero, P., Minetti, B., Comotti, B., Bassan, R., and Barbui, T. (1985). Danazol for the treatment of idiopathic thrombocytopaenic purpura. *Acta Haematologia*, **74**, 97–8.

Bunn, P. A., Foon, K. A., Ihde, D. C., Longo, D. L., Eddy, J., Winkler, C. F. *et al.* (1984). Recombinant leukocyte A interferon: An active agent in advanced cutaneous T-cell lymphomas. *Annals of Internal Medicine*, **101**, 484–7.

Buzdar, A. U., Blumenschein, G. R., Smith, T. L., Powell, K. C., Hortobagyi, G. N., Yap, H. Y. *et al.* (1984). Adjuvant chemotherapy with fluorouracil, doxorubicin and cyclophosphamide, with or without Bacillus Calmette–Guerin and with or without irradiation in operable breast cancer. *Cancer*, **53**, 384–9.

Campbell, R. C. (1989). *Statistics for biologists*, 3rd edn. Cambridge University Press, Cambridge.

Cannon, G. W., Pincus, S. H., Emkey, R. D., Denes, A., Cohen, S. A., Wolfe, F., *et al.* (1989). Double-blind trial of recombinant gamma-interferon versus placebo in the treatment of rheumatoid arthritis. *Arthritis and Rheumatism*, **32**, 964–73.

Carter, W. A., Strayer, D. R., Brodsky, I., Lewin, M., Pellegrino, M. G., Einck, L. *et al.* (1987). Clinical, immunological and virological effects of ampligen, a mismatched double-stranded RNA, in patients with AIDS or AIDS-related complex. *Lancet*, **i**, 1286–92.

CDC (1986). Centers for Disease Control classification system for human T-lymphotrophic virus type III/lymphadenopathy associated virus infections. *MMWR*, **35**, 334–9.

Christensen, E. (1987). Multivariate survival analysis using Cox's regression model. *Hepatology*, **7**, 1346–58.

Clemens, J. D., Sack, D. A., Harris, J. R., Chakraborty, J., Khan, M. R., Stanton, B. F. *et al.* (1988). Impact of B subunit killed whole-cell and killed whole-cell-only oral vaccines against cholera upon treated diarrhoeal illness and mortality in an area endemic for cholera. *Lancet*, **i**, 1375–9.

Cohen, A. S., Reynolds, W. E., Franklin, E. C., Kulka, J. P., Ropes, M. W., Shulman, L. E. *et al.* (1971). Preliminary criteria for the classification of systemic lupus erythematosus. *Bulletin on the Rheumatic Diseases*, **21**, 643–8.

Corrado, O. J., Pastorello, E., Ollier, S., Cresswell, L., Zanussi, C., Ortolani, C. *et al.* (1989). A double-blind study of hyposensitisation with an alginate conjugated extract of *D. pteronyssinus* (Conjuvac[R]) in patients with perennial rhinitis. *Allergy*, **44**, 108–15.

Coutinho, R. A., Lelie, P. N., Albrecht-van Lent, P., Reerink-Brongers, E. E., Stoutjesdijk, L., Dees, P. *et al.* (1983). Efficacy of a heat inactivated hepatitis B vaccine in male homosexuals: outcome of a placebo controlled double blind trial. *British Medical Journal*, **286**, 1305–8.

Creagan, E. T., Buckner, J. C., Hahn, R. G., Richardson, R. R., Schaid, D. J., and Kovach, J. S. (1988). An evaluation of recombinant leukocyte A interferon with aspirin in patients with metastatic renal cell cancer. *Cancer*, **61**, 1787–91.

Crispe, I. N. (1988). Mechanisms of self-tolerance. *Immunology Today*, **9**, 329–31.

Crosnier, J., Jungers, P., Courouce, A-M., Laplanche, A., Benhamou, E., Degos, F. *et al.* (1981). Randomised placebo-controlled trial of hepatitis B surface antigen vaccine in French haemodialysis units: 1, Medical staff. *Lancet*, **i**, 455–9.

Davis, S., Mietlowski, W., Rohwedder, J. J., Griffin, J. P., and Neshat, A. A. (1982). Levamisole as an adjuvant to chemotherapy in extensive broncho-genic carcinoma. *Cancer*, **50**, 646–51.

de Weck, A. (1985). New approaches to desensitisation in IgE-mediated allergy. *Clinics in Immunology and Allergy*, **5**, 1–11.

de Wit, R., Schattenkerk, J. K. M. E., Boucher, C. A. B., Bakker, P. J. M., Veenhof, K. H. N., and Danner, S. A. (1988). Clinical and virological effects of high-dose recombinant interferon-alpha in disseminated AIDS-related Kaposi's sarcoma. *Lancet*, **ii**, 1214–7.

de Wolf, F., Goudsmit, J., Paul, D. A., Lange, J. M. A., Hooijkaas, C., Shellekens, P. *et al.* (1987). Risk of AIDS-related complex and AIDS in homosexual men with persistent HIV antigenaemia. *British Medical Journal*, **295**, 569–72.

Dooley, J. S., Davis, G. L., Peters, M., Waggoner, J. G., Goodman, Z., and Hoofnagle, J. H. (1986). Pilot study of recombinant human alpha-interferon for chronic type B hepatitis. *Gastroenterology*, **90**, 150–7.

Dorval, T., Palangie, T., Jouve, M., Garcia-Giralt, E., Israel, L. Falcoff, E. *et al.* (1986). Clinical phase II trial of recombinant DNA interferon (interferon alfa 2b) in patients with metastatic malignant melanoma. *Cancer*, **58**, 215–8.

Dougados, M., Awada, H., and Amor, B. (1988). Cyclosporin in rheumatoid arthritis: a double-blind, placebo controlled study in 52 patients. *Annals of the Rheumatic Diseases*, **47**, 127–33.

Dupre, J., Stiller, C. R., Kolb, H., von Graffenried, B., Gent, M., Nerup, J. *et al.* (The Canadian-European Randomised Control Trial Group) (1988). Cyclosporin-induced remission of IDDM after early intervention. *Diabetes*, **37**, 1574–82.

DuRant, R. H., Dyken, P. R., and Swift, A. V. (1982). The influence of inosiplex treatment on the neurological disability of patients with subacute sclerosing panencephalitis. *Journal of Paediatrics*, **101**, 288–93.

Ellis, C. N., Gorsulowsky, D. C., Hamilton, T. A., Billings, J. K., Brown, M. D., Headington, J. T. *et al.* (1986). Cyclosporine improves psoriasis in a double-blind study. *Journal of the American Medical Association*, **256**, 3110–6.

Eriksson, B., Oberg, K., Alm, G., Karlsson, A., Lundqvist, G., Andersson, T. *et al.* (1986). Treatment of malignant endocrine pancreatic tumours with human leucocyte interferon. *Lancet*, **ii**, 1307–9.

Eron, L. J., Judson, F., Tucker, S., Prawer, S., Mills, J., Murphy, K. *et al.* (1986). Interferon therapy for *Condylomata acuminata*. *New England Journal of Medicine*, **315**, 1059–64.

Evans, S. J. W., Mills, P., and Dawson, J. (1988). The end of the p-value? *British Heart Journal*, **60**, 177–80.

Ewan, P. W., Alexander, M. M., Snape, C., Ind, P. W., Agrell, B., and Dreborg, S. (1988). Effective hyposensitisation in allergic rhinitis using a potent partially purified extract of house dust mite. *Clinical Allergy*, **18**, 501–8.

Fagan, E. A. and Eddlestone, A. L. W. F. (1985). Hepatitis vaccination. *Clinics in Immunology and Allergy*, **5**, 43–85.

Farr, B. M., Gwaltney, J. M., Adams, K. F., and Hayden, F. G. (1984). Intranasal interferon alpha-2 for prevention of natural rhinovirus colds. *Antimicrobial Agents and Chemotherapy*, **26**, 31–4.

Feutren, G., Papoz, L., Assan, R., Vialettes, B., Karsenty, G., Vexiau, P. *et al.* (1986). Cyclosporin increases the rate and length of remissions in insulin-dependent diabetes of recent onset. *Lancet*, **ii**, 119–24.

Feutren, G., Querin, S., Noel, L. H., Chatenoud, L., Beaurain, G., Tron, F. *et al.* (1987). Effects of cyclosporine in severe systemic lupus erythematosus. *Journal of Paediatrics*, **111**, 1063–8.

Fisher, R. I., Coltman, C. A., Doroshow, J. H., Rayner, A. A., Hawkins, M. J., Mier, J. W. *et al.* (1988). Metastatic renal cancer treated with interleukin-2 and lymphokine-activated killer cells: A phase II clinical trial. *Annals of Internal Medicine*, **108**, 518–23.

Flores, J., Perez-Schael, I., Gonzalez, M., Garcia, D., Perez, M., Daoud, N. *et al.* (1987). Protection against severe rotavirus diarrhoea by rhesus rotavirus vaccine in Venezualan infants. *Lancet*, **i**, 882–4.

Foon, K. A., Shwerwin, S. A., Abrams, P. G., Longo, D. L., Fer, M. F., Stevenson, H. C. *et al.* (1984). Treatment of advanced non-Hodgkin's lymphoma with recombinant leukocyte A interferon. *New England Journal of Medicine*, **311**, 1148–52.

Fox, R. M., Woods, R. L., Tattersall, M. H. N., and Basten, A. (1980). A randomised study of adjuvant immunotherapy with levamisole and *Corynebacterium parvum* in operable non-small cell lung cancer. *International Journal of Radiation Oncology, Biology and Physics*, **6**, 1043–5.

Francis, D. P., Hadler, S. C., Thompson, S. E., Maynard, J. E., Ostrow, D. G., Altman, N. *et al.* (1982). The prevention of Hepatitis B with vaccine: report of the Centers for Disease Control multi-center efficacy trial among homosexual men. *Annals of Internal Medicine*, **97**, 362–6.

Frediksson, T. and Petterson, V. (1978). Severe psoriasis: oral therapy with a new retinoid. *Dermatologica*, **157**, 238–44.

Freedman, L. S. (1982). Tables of numbers of patients required in clinical trials using the logrank test. *Statistics in Medicine*, **1**, 121–9.

Furst, D. E. (1988). Clinical evaluation of drugs in rheumatoid arthritis. *Advances in Inflammation Research*, **12**, 227–38.

Gabrilove, J. L., Jakubowski, A., Scher, H., Sternberg, C., Wong, G., Grous, J. *et al.* (1988). Effect of granulocyte colony stimulating factor on neutropaenia and associated morbidity due to chemotherapy for transitional-cell carcinoma of the urothelium. *New England Journal of Medicine*, **318**, 1414–22.

Gardner, M. J. and Altman, D. G. (1986). Confidence intervals rather than P values: estimation rather than hypothesis testing. *British Medical Journal*, **292**, 746–50.

Geffen, J. R., Klein, R. J., and Friedman-Kien, A. E. (1984). Intralesional administration of large doses of human leukocyte interferon for the treatment of *Condylomata acuminata*. *Journal of Infectious Diseases*, **150**, 612–5.

Gehan, E. A. (1965). A generalised Wilcoxon test for comparing arbitrarily singly-censored samples. *Biometrika*, **52**, 203–23.

Gibson, J. R. and Harvey, S. G. (1984). Interferon in the treatment of persistant viral warts. *Dermatologica*, **169**, 47–8.

Giles, F. J., Singer, C. R. J., Gray, A. G., Yong, K. L., Brozovic, M., Davies, S. C. *et al.* (1988). Alpha interferon therapy for essential thrombocythaemia. *Lancet*, **ii**, 70–2.

Giuliano, A. E., Sparks, F. C., Patterson, K., Spears, I., and Morton, D. L. (1986). Adjuvant chemo-immunotherapy in stage II carcinoma of the breast. *Journal of Surgical Oncology*, **31**, 255–9.

Giustolisi, R., Guglielmo, P., Cacciola, E., and Cacciola, R. R. (1983). Thymostimulin in aplastic anaemia. *Acta Haematologia*, **69**, 417–8.

Golumb, H. M., Ratain, M. J., Fefer, A., Thompson, J., Golde, D. W., Ozer, H. *et al.* (1988). Randomised study of the duration of treatment with interferon alpha-2B in patients with hairy cell leukaemia. *Journal of the National Cancer Institute*, **80**, 369–73.

Grammer, L. C., Shaughnessy, M. A., Bernhard, M. I., Finkle, S. M., Pyle, H. R., Silvestri, L. *et al.* (1987). The safety and activity of polymerised ragweed: a double-blind placebo-controlled trial in 81 patients with ragweed rhinitis. *Journal of Allergy and Clinical Immunology*, **80**, 177–83.

Gray, B. N., Walker, C., Andrewartha, L., Freeman, S., and Bennett, R. C. (1989). Controlled clinical trial of adjuvant immunotherapy with BCG and neuraminidase-treated autologous tumour cells in large bowel cancer. *Journal of Surgical Oncology*, **40**, 34–7.

Groopman, J. E., Gottlieb, M. S., Goodman, J., Mitsuyasu, R. T., Conant, M. A., Prince, H. *et al.* (1984). Recombinant alpha-2 Interferon therapy for Kaposi's sarcoma associated with the acquired immunodeficiency syndrome. *Annals of Internal Medicine*, **100**, 671–6.

Groopman, J. E., Mitsuyasu, R. T., DeLeo, M. J., Oette, D. H., and Golde, D. W. (1987). Effect of recombinant human granulocyte-macrophage colony stimulating factor on myelopoiesis in the acquired immunodeficiency syndrome. *New England Journal of Medicine*, **317**, 593–8.

Gutterman, J. U., Blumenschein, G. R., Alexanian, R., Yap, H-Y., Buzdar,

A. U., Cabanillas, F. *et al.* (1980). Leukocyte interferon-induced tumour regression in human metastatic breast cancer, multiple myeloma and malignant lymphoma. *Annals of Internal Medicine*, **93**, 399–406.

Hanlon, P., Hanlon, L., Marsh, V., Byass, P., Shenton, F., Hassan-King, M. *et al.* (1987). Trial of an attenuated bovine rotavirus vaccine (RIT 4237) in Gambian infants. *Lancet*, **i**, 1342–5.

Haque, K. N. and Zaidi, M. H. (1988). IgM-enriched intravenous immunoglobulin therapy in neonatal sepsis. *American Journal of Diseases in Childhood*, **142**, 1293–6.

Hayat, M., Jehn, U. Willemze, R., Haanen, C., Zittoun, R., Monconduit, M. *et al.* (1986). A randomised comparison of maintenance treatment with androgens, immunotherapy and chemotherapy in adult acute myelogenous leukaemia. *Cancer*, **58**, 617–23.

Hazelton, R. A., McCruden, A. B., Sturrock, R. D., and Stimson, W. H. (1983). Hormonal manipulation of the immune response in systemic lupus erythematosus: a drug trial of an anabolic steroid, 19-nortestosterone. *Annals of the Rheumatic Diseases*, **42**, 155–7.

Hess, A. D., Esa, A. H., and Colombani, P. M. (1988). Mechanisms of action of cyclosporine: effect on cells of the immune system and on subcellular events in T-cell activation. *Transplantation Proceedings*, XX (2 supplement 2), 29–40.

Higgins, P. G., Phillpotts, R. J., Scott, G. M., Wallace, J., Bernhardt, L. L., and Tyrell, D. A. J. (1983). Intranasal Interferon as protection against experimental respiratory Coronavirus infection in volunteers. *Antimicrobial Agents and Chemotherapy*, **24**, 713–5.

Himmelweit, F. and Marquardt, M. (eds) (1956). *The collected papers of Paul Ehrlich*. Pergamon Press, London.

Hirsch, M. S., Schooley, R. T., Cosimi, A. B., Russell, P. S., Delmonico, F. L., Tolkoff-Rubin, N. E. *et al.* (1983). Effects of interferon-alpha on cytomegalovirus reactivation syndromes in renal-transplant recipients. *New England Journal of Medicine*, **308**, 1489–93.

Hoke, C. H., Nisalak, A., Sangawhipa, N., Jatanasen, S., Laorakapongse, T., Innis, B. L. *et al.* (1988). Protection against Japanese encephalitis by inactivated vaccines. *New England Journal of Medicine*, **319**, 608–14.

Hubay, C. A., Pearson, O. H., Mann, A., Gordon, N. H., and McGuire, W. L. (1985). Adjuvant endocrine therapy, cytotoxic chemotherapy and immunotherapy in stage II breast cancer: 6-year result. *Journal of Steroid Biochemistry*, **23**, 1147–50.

Humphrey, L. J., Taschier-Collins, S., and Volenec, F. J. (1984). Treatment of primary breast cancer with immunotherapy: comparison with adjuvant chemotherapy and radiation therapy. *American Journal of Surgery*, **148**, 649–52.

Ikic, D., Krusic, J., Kirhmajer, V., Knezevic, M., Maricic, Z., Rode, B. *et al.* (1981). Application of human leucocyte interferon in patients with carcinoma of the uterine cervix. *Lancet*, **i**, 1027–30.

Imbach, P., Barandun, S., Baumgartner, C., Hirt, A., Hofer, F., and Wagner,

H. P. (1981a). High-dose intravenous gammaglobulin therapy of refractory, in particular idiopathic thrombocytopaenia in childhood. *Helvetica Paediatrica Acta*, **46**, 81–6.

Imbach, P., Barandun, S., d'Apuzzo, V., Baumgartner, C., Hirt, A., Morell, A. *et al.* (1981b). High-dose intravenous gammaglobulin for idiopathic thrombocytopaenic purpura in childhood. *Lancet*, **i**, 1228–31.

Isenberg, D. A., Snaith, M. L., Morrow, W. J. W., Al-Khader, A. A., Cohen, S. L., Fischer, C. *et al.* (1981). Cyclosporin A for the treatment of systemic lupus erythematosus. *International Journal of Immunopharmacology*, **3**, 163–9.

Jackson, G. G., Perkins, J. T., Rubenis, M., Paul, D. A., Knigge, M., Despotes, J. C. *et al.* (1988). Passive immunoneutralisation of human immunodeficiency virus in patients with advanced AIDS. *Lancet*, **ii**, 647–52.

Jacobs, A. D., Champlin, R. E., and Golde, D. W. (1985). Recombinant alpha$_2$ interferon for hairy cell leukaemia. *Blood*, **65**, 1017–20.

Jacobs, L., O'Malley, J., Freeman, A., Murawski, J., and Ekes, R. (1982). Intrathecal interferon in multiple sclerosis. *Archives of Neurology*, **39**, 609–15.

Jones, C. E., Dyken, P. R., Huttenlocher, P. R., Jarbour, J. T., and Maxwell, K. W. (1982). Inosiplex therapy in subacute sclerosing panencephalitis. *Lancet*, **i**, 1034–7.

Jones, J. V. (1985). Plasmapheresis. *Clinics in Immunology and Allergy*, **5**, 13–32.

Jungers, P., Kuttenn, F., Liote, F., Pelissier, C., Athea, N., Laurent, M-C. *et al.* (1985). Hormonal modulation in systemic lupus erythematosus. *Arthritis and Rheumatism*, **28**, 1243–50.

Kalimo, K. O. K., Joronen, I. A., and Havu, V. K. (1983). Failure of oral inosiplex treatment of recurrent herpes simplex virus infections. *Archives of Dermatology*, **119**, 463–7.

Kantharia, B. K., Goulding, N. J., Hall, N. D., Davies, J., Maddison, P. J., Bacon, P. A. *et al.* (1989). Thymopentin (TP-5) in the treatment of rheumatoid arthritis. *British Journal of Rheumatology*, **28**, 118–23.

Khoo, S. K., Whitaker, S. V., Jones, I. S. C., and Thomas, D. A. (1984). Levamisole as adjuvant to chemotherapy of ovarian cancer: results of a randomised trial and 4-year follow up. *Cancer*, **54**, 986–90.

Kinsella, P. L., Ebringer, R. W., and Corbett, M. (1980). Levamisole in rheumatoid arthritis—a double-blind study. *Journal of Rheumatology*, **7**, 288–92.

Kirkwood, J. M., Ernstoff, M. S., Davis, C. A., Reiss, M., Ferraresi, R., and Rudnick, S. A. (1985a). Comparison of intramuscular and intravenous recombinant alpha$_2$ interferon in melanoma and other cancers. *Annals of Internal Medicine*, **103**, 32–6.

Kirkwood, J. M., Harris, J. E., Vera, R., Sandler, S., Fischer, D. S., Khandekar, J. *et al.* (1985b). A randomised study of low and high doses of leukocyte alpha-interferon in metastatic renal cell carcinoma: the American Cancer Society Collaborative Trial. *Cancer Research*, **45**, 863–71.

Klatzmann, D. and Gluckman, J. C. (1986). HIV infection: facts and hypotheses. *Immunology Today*, **7**, 291–6.

Knobler, R. L., Panitch, H. S., Braheny, S. L., Sipe, J. C., Rice, G. P. A., Huddlestone, J. R. *et al.* (1984). Systemic alpha-interferon therapy of multiple sclerosis. *Neurology*, **34**, 1273–9.

Kovacs, J. A., Deyton, L., Davey, R., Falloon, J., Zunich, K., Lee, D., *et al.* (1989). Combined zidovudine and interferon-alpha therapy in patients with Kaposi sarcoma and AIDS. *Annals of Internal Medicine*, **111**, 280–7.

Koyama, S., Ozaki, A., Iwasaki, Y., Sakita, T., Osuga, T., Watanabe, A. *et al.* (1986). Randomised controlled study of postoperative adjuvant immunochemotherapy with *Nocardia rubra* cell wall skelton (N-CWS) and Tegafur for gastric carcinoma. *Cancer Immunology and Immunotherapy*, **22**, 148–54.

Krown, S. E., Real, F. X., Cunningham-Rundles, S., Myskowski, P. L., Koziner, B., Fein, S. *et al.* (1983). Preliminary observations on the effect of recombinant leukocyte A interferon in homosexual men with Kaposi's sarcoma. *New England Journal of Medicine*, **308**, 1071–6.

Kurtzke, J. F. (1965). Further notes on disability evaluation in multiple sclerosis, with scale modifications. *Neurology*, **15**, 654–61.

Lachmann, P. J., Grant, R. M., Freedman, L. S., Sikora, K., and Bleehen, N. M. (1985). A preliminary trial of a novel form of active immunotherapy in squamous cell carcinoma of the lung. *British Journal of Cancer*, **51**, 415–7.

Lai, K. N., Lai, F. M-M., and Vallence-Owen, J. (1988). A short-term controlled trial of cyclosporin A in IgA nephropathy. *Transplantation proceedings*, **XX** (3 supplement 4), 297–303.

Lang, J. M., Touraine, J-L., Trepo, C., Choutet, P., Kirstetter, M., Falkenrodt, A. *et al.* (1988). Randomised, double-blind, placebo-controlled trial of ditiocarb sodium ('imuthiol') in human immunodeficiency virus infection. *Lancet*, **ii**, 702–6.

Langman, M. J. S. (1986). Towards estimation and confidence intervals. *British Medical Journal*, **292**, 716.

Leahy, B. C., Honeybourne, D., Brear, S. G., Carroll, K. B., Thatcher, N., and Stretton, T. B. (1985). Treatment of malignant pleural effusions with intrapleural *Corynebacterium parvum* or tetracycline. *European Journal of Respiratory Diseases*, **66**, 50–4.

Lenhard, R. E., Order, S. E., Spunberg, J. J., Asbell, S. O., and Leibel, S. A. (1985). Isotopic immunoglobulin: a new systemic therapy for advanced Hodgkin's disease. *Journal of Clinical Oncolcogy*, **3**, 1296–300.

Lessner, H. E., Mayer, R. J., Ellenberg, S. S., Holyoke, E. D., Moertel, C. G., O'Connell, M. J. *et al.* (The Gastrointestinal Tumour Study Group) (1984). Adjuvant therapy of colon cancer—results of a prospectively randomised trial. *New England Journal of Medicine*, **310**, 737–43.

Lotze, M. T., Custer, M. C., and Rosenberg, S. A. (1986). Intraperitoneal administration of interleukin-2 in patients with cancer. *Archives of Surgery*, **121**, 1373–9.

Lotz, M. and Vaughan, J. H. (1988). Rheumatoid arthritis. In: *Immunological diseases* (ed. M. Samter., D. W. Talmage., M. M. Frank., K. F. Austen and H. N. Claman, vol. II, pp. 1365–1416 Little Brown, Boston, USA.

Malling, H-J., Dreborg, S., and Weeke, B. (1986). Diagnosis and immunotherapy of mould allergy: V. Clinical efficacy and side-effects of immunotherapy with *Cladosporium herbarum*. *Allergy*, **41**, 507–19.

Mandelli, F., Tribalto, M., Avvisati, G., Cantonetti, M., Petrucci, M. T., Boccadoro, M. *et al.* (1988). Recombinant interferon alfa-2b (INTRON A) as a post-induction therapy for responding multiple myeloma patients. M84 protocol. *Cancer Treatment Reviews*, 15 (Supplement A), 43–8.

Marget, W., Mar, P. J., Jaspers, L., Possinger, K., and Haslberger, H. (1985). Preliminary study on administration of high-titer lipid A antibody serum in sepsis and septic shock patients. *Infection*, **13**, 120–4.

Marks, J. G., Trautlein, J. J., Epstein, W. L., Laws, D. M., and Sicard, G. R. (1987). Oral hyposensitisation to poison ivy and poison oak. *Archives of Dermatology*, **123**, 476–8.

Maupas, P., Chiron, J-P., Barin, F., Coursaget, P., Goudeau, A., Perrin, J. *et al.* (1981). Efficacy of a hepatitis B vaccine in prevention of early HBsAg carrier state in children: controlled trial in an endemic area (Senegal). *Lancet*, **i**, 289–92.

Maver, C., Kausel, H., Lininger, L., and McKneally, M. (1982). Intrapleural BCG immunotherapy of lung cancer patients. *Recent Results in Cancer Research*, **80**, 227–31.

McCabe, B. F., and Clark, K. F. (1983). Interferon and laryngeal papillomatosis: the Iowa experience. *Annals of Otology, Rhinology and Laryngology*, **92**, 2–7.

McDonald, W. I. and Halliday, A. M. (1977). Diagnosis and classification of multiple sclerosis. *British Medical Bulletin*, **3**, 4–9.

Meeker, T. C., Lowder, J., Malony, D. G., Miller, R. A., Thielemans, K., Warnke, R. *et al.* (1985). A clinical trial of anti-idiotype therapy for B cell malignancy. *Blood*, **65**, 1349–63.

Merchant, R. E., Grant, A. J., Merchant, L. H., and Young, H. F. (1988). Adoptive immunotherapy for recurrent glioblastoma multiforme using lymphokine-activated killer cells and recombinant interleukin-2. *Cancer*, **62**, 665–71.

Meyers, J. D., McGuffin, R. W., Neiman, P. E., Singer, J. W., and Thomas, E. D. (1980). Toxicity and efficacy of human leukocyte interferon for treatment of cytomegalovirus pneumonia after marrow transplantation. *Journal of Infectious Diseases*, **141**, 555–62.

Meyers, J. D., McGuffin, R. W., Bryson, Y. J., Cantell, K., and Thomas, E. D. (1982). Treatment of cytomegalovirus pneumonia after marrow transplant with combined vidarabine and human leukocyte interferon. *Journal of Infectious Diseases*, **146**, 80–4.

Meyers, J. D., Leszczynski, J., Zaia, J. A., Flournoy, N., Newton, B., Snydman, D. R. *et al.* (1983). Prevention of cytomegalovirus infection by cytomegalovirus immune globulin after marrow transplantation. *Annals of Internal Medicine*, **98**, 442–6.

Miller, B., De Merieux, P., Srinivasan, R., Clements, P., Fan, P., Levy, J. *et al.* (1980). Double-blind placebo controlled crossover evaluation of levamisole in rheumatoid arthritis. *Arthritis and Rheumatism*, **23**, 172–82.

Moller, C., Bjorksten, B., Nilsson, B., and Dreborg, S. (1984). The precision of the conjunctival provocation test. *Allergy*, **39**, 37–41.

Moller, C., Dreborg, S., Lanner, A., and Bjorksten, B. (1986). Oral immunotherapy of children with Rhinoconjunctivitis due to birch pollen allergy. *Allergy*, **41**, 271–9.

Morgan, S. H. and Hughes, G. R. V. (1985). The laboratory investigation of rheumatic and connective tissue diseases. *Clinics in Immunology and Allergy*, **5**, 513–30.

Moss, A. R., Bacchetti, P., Osmond, D., Krampf, W., Chaisson, R. E., Stites, D. *et al.* (1988). Seropositivity for HIV and the development of AIDS or AIDS-related conditions: three year follow-up of the San Francisco General Hospital cohort. *British Medical Journal*, **296**, 745–50.

Movat, H. Z. (1985). *The inflammatory reaction.* Elsevier, Amsterdam.

Mowat, A. G. and Mowat, A. M. (1981). Levamisole in rheumatoid arthritis: a comparison with D-penicillamine. *Journal of Rheumatology*, **8**, 575–80.

Muller U., Rabson, A. R., Bischof, M., Lomnitzer, R., Dreborg, S., and Lanner, A. (1987). A double-blind study comparing monomethoxy polyethylene glycol-modified honeybee venom and unmodified honeybee venom for immunotherapy. *Journal of Allergy and Clinical Immunology*, **80**, 252–61.

Muss, H. B., Welander, C., Caponera, M., Reavis, K., Cruz, J. M., Cooper, R. *et al.* (1985). Interferon and doxorubicin in renal cell carcinoma. *Cancer Treatment Reports*, **69**, 721–2.

Neifeld, J. P., Terz, J. J., Kaplan, A. M., and Lawrence, W. Jr. (1985). Adjuvant *Corynebacterium parvum* immunotherapy for squamous cell epitheliomas of the oral cavity, pharynx and larynx. *Journal of Surgical Oncology*, **28**, 137–45.

Nemunaitis, J., Singer, J. W., Buckner, D., Hill, R., Storb, R., Thomas, E. D. *et al.* (1988). Use of recombinant human granulocyte-macrophage colony stimulating factor in autologous bone-marrow transplantation for lymphoid malignancies. *Blood*, **72**, 834–6.

Newland, A. C., Treleaven, J. G., Minchinton, R. M., and Waters, A. H. (1983). High-dose intravenous IgG in adults with autoimmune thrombocytopaenia. *Lancet*, **i**, 84–7.

Noon, L. (1911). Prophylactic inoculation against hayfever. *Lancet*, **i**, 1572–3.

Nussenblat, R. B., Palestine, A. G., Rook, A. H., Scher, I., Wacker, W. B., and Gery, I. (1983*a*). Treatment of intraocular inflammatory disease with cyclosporin A. *Lancet*, **ii**, 235–8.

Nussenblat, R. B., Palestine, A. G., and Chan, C-C. (1983*b*). Cyclosporin A therapy in the treatment of intraocular inflammatory disease resistant to systemic corticosteroids and cytotoxic agents. *American Journal of Ophthalmology*, **96**, 275–82.

Oberg, K., Funa, K., and Alm, G. (1983). Effects of leukocyte interferon on clinical symptoms and hormone levels in patients with mid-gut carcinoid tumours and carcinoid syndrome. *New England Journal of Medicine*, **309**, 129–33.

Oberg, K., Norheim, I., Lind, E., Alm, G., Lundqvist, G., Wide, L. *et al.* (1986). Treatment of malignant carcinoid tumours with human leucocyte interferon: long-term results. *Cancer Treatment Reports*, **70**, 1297–304.

Ochiai, T., Sato, H., Hayashi, R., Asano, T., Sato, H., and Yamamura, Y. (1983). Postoperative adjuvant immunotherapy of gastric cancer with BCG-cell wall skeleton: 3- to 6-year follow up of a randomised clinical trial. *Cancer Immunology and Immunotherapy*, **14**, 167–71.

Ohman, J. L., Findlay, S. R., and Leitermann, K. M. (1984). Immunotherapy in cat-induced asthma. Double-blind trial with evaluation of *in vivo* and *in vitro* responses. *Journal of Allergy and Clinical Immunology*, **74**, 230–9.

Omura, G. A., Vogler, W. R., Lefante, J., Silberman, H., Knopse, W., Gordon, D. *et al.* (1982). Treatment of acute myelogenous leukaemia: influence of three induction regimens and maintenance with chemotherapy or BCG immunotherapy. *Cancer*, **49**, 1530–6.

Onji, M., Kondoh, H., Horiike, N., Yamaguchi, S., Ogawa, Y., Kumon, I., *et al.* (1987). Effect of recombinant interleukin-2 on hepatitis B e antigen positive chronic hepatitis. *Gut*, **28**, 1648–52.

Order, S. E., Stillwagon, G. B., Klein, J. L., Leichner, P. K., Siegelman, S. S., Fishman, E. K. *et al.* (1985). Iodine 131 antiferritin, a new modality in hepatoma: A Radiation Therapy Oncology Group Study. *Journal of Clinical Oncology*, **3**, 1573–82.

O'Reilly, R. J. O., Reich, L., Gold, J., Kirkpatrick, D., Dinsmore, R., Kapoor, N. *et al.* (1983). A randomised trial of intravenous hyperimmune globulin for the prevention of cytomegalovirus (CMV) infections following marrow transplantation. Preliminary results. *Transplantation Proceedings*, **XV**, 1405–11.

Orholm, M., Pedersen, C., Mathiesen, L., Dowd, P., and Nielsen, J. O. (1989). Suppression of p24 antigen in sera from HIV-infected individuals with low-dose alpha-interferon and zidovudine. A pilot study. *AIDS*, **3**, 97–100.

Ortolani, C., Pastorello, E., Moss, R. B., Hsu, Y-P., Restuccia, M., Joppolo, G. *et al.* (1984). Grass pollen immunotherapy: a single year double-blind, placebo-controlled study in patients with grass pollen-induced asthma and rhinitis. *Journal of Allergy and Clinical Immunology*, **73**, 283–90.

Ota, K., Kurita, S., Yamada, K., Masaoka, T., Uzuka, Y., and Ogawa, N. (1986). Immunotherapy with bestatin for acute nonlymphocytic leukaemia in adults. *Cancer Immunology and Immunotherapy*, **23**, 5–10.

Ottesen, E. and Sher, A. (1988). Immunoparasitology. In: *Immunological diseases* (eds M. Samter, D. W. Talmage, M. M. Frank, K. F., Austin, and H. N. Claman, vol. I, pp. 923–44. Little, Brown, Boston, USA.

Palmisano, L., Chisesi, T., Galli, M., Gritti, F. M., Ielasi, G., Lazzarin, A. *et al.* (1988). Thymostimulin treatment in AIDS-related complex. *Clinical Immunology and Immunopathology*, **47**, 253–61.

Palmovic, D. (1987). Prevention of hepatitis B infection in health care workers after accidental exposure. *Journal of Infection*, **15**, 221–4.

Perrillo, R. P., Regenstein, F. G., Peters, M. G., DeSchryver-Kecskemeti, K., Bodicky, C. J., Campbell, C. R. *et al.* (1988). Prednisone withdrawal followed by recombinant alpha interferon in the treatment of chronic type B hepatitis. *Annals of Internal Medicine*, **109**, 95–100.

Pestka, S., Langer, J. A., Zoon, K. C., and Samuel, C. E. (1987). Interferons and their actions. *Annual Review of Biochemistry*, **56**, 727–77.

Plotkin, S. A., Smiley, M. L., Friedman, H. M., Starr, S. E., Fleisher, G. R., Wlodaver, C. *et al.* (1984). Towne-vaccine-induced prevention of cytomegalovirus disease after renal transplants. *Lancet*, **i**, 528–30.

Pocock, S. J. (1983). *Clinical trials: a practical approach*. Wiley, New York.

Pocock, S. J. and Simon, R. (1975). Sequential treatment assignment with balancing for prognostic factors in the controlled clinical trial. *Biometrics*, **31**, 103–16.

Pocock, S. J., Hughes, M. D., and Lee, R. J. (1987). Statistical problems in the reporting of clinical trials. *New England Journal of Medicine*, **317**, 426–32.

Poser, C. M., Paty, D. W., and Scheinberg, L. C. (1983). New diagnostic criteria for multiple sclerosis: guidelines for research protocols. *Annals of Neurology*, **13**, 227–31.

Price, J. F., Warner, J. O., Hey, E. N., Turner, M. W., and Soothill, J. F. (1984). A controlled trial of hyposensitisation with adsorbed tyrosine *Dermatophagoides pteronyssinus* antigen in childhood asthma: *in vivo* aspects. *Clinical Allergy*, **14**, 209–19.

Quesada, J. R., Hersh, E. M., Keating, M., Zander, A., and Hester, J. (1981). Hairy cell leukaemia: clinical effects of the methanol extraction residue (MER) of BCG, lithium carbonate and mononuclear cell-enriched leukocyte transfusions. *Leukaemia Research*, **5**, 463–76.

Quesada, J. R., Reuben, J., Manning J. T., Hersh, E. M., and Gutterman, J. U. (1984). Alpha-interferon for induction of remission in hairy cell leukaemia. *New England Journal of Medicine*, **310**, 15–18.

Quesada, J. R., Hersh, E. M., Manning, J., Reuben, J., Keating M., Schnipper, E. *et al.* (1986a). Treatment of Hairy Cell Leukaemia with recombinant alpha-interferon. *Blood*, **68**, 493–7.

Quesada, J. R., Alexanian, R., Hawkins, M., Barlogie, B., Borden, E., Itri, L. *et al.* (1986b). Treatment of multiple myeloma with recombinant alpha-interferon. *Blood*, **67**, 275–8.

Rambaldi, A., Introna, M., Colotta, F., Landolfo, S., Colombo, N., Mangioni, C. *et al.* (1985). Intraperitoneal administration of interferon-beta in ovarian cancer patients. *Cancer*, **56**, 294–301.

Ratain, M. J., Golumb, H. M., Vardiman, J. W., Vokes, E. E., Jacobs, R. H., and Daly, K. (1985). Treatment of hairy cell leukaemia with recombinant alpha$_2$ interferon. *Blood*, **65**, 644–8.

Reilly, S., Dhillon, B. J., Nkanza, K. M., D'Souza, A., Taylor, N., Hobbs, S. *et al.* (1986). Adenovirus type 8 keratoconjunctivitis—an outbreak and its treatment with topical human fibroblast interferon. *Journal of hygiene (Cambridge)*, **96**, 557–75.

Ritchie, D. M., Boyle, J. A., McInnes, J. M., Jasani, M. K., Dalakos, T. G., Grieveson, P. *et al.* (1968). Clinical studies with an articular index for the assessment of joint tenderness in patients with rheumatoid arthritis. *Quarterly Journal of Medicine*, **XXXVII**, 393–406.

Ropes, M. W., Bennet, G. A., Cobb, S., Jacox, R., and Jessar, R. A. (1958). 1958 revision of diagnostic criteria for Rheumatoid Arthritis. *Bulletin on the Rheumatic Diseases*, **9**, 175–6.

Ropes, M. W. (1959). Diagnostic criteria for rheumatoid arthritis. 1958 revision. *Annals of the Rheumatic Diseases*, **18**, 49–53.

Rosenberg, S. A., Lotze, M. T., Muul, L. M., Chang, A. E., Avis, F. P., Leitman, S. *et al.* (1987). Progress report on the treatment of 157 patients with advanced cancer using lymphokine-activated killer cells and interleukin-2 or high-dose interleukin-2 alone. *New England Journal of Medicine*, **316**, 889–97.

Roszkowski, K., Nozaryn-Plotnicki, B., Roszkowski, W., Ko, H. L., Jeljaszewicz, J., and Pulverer, G. (1985). Small-cell lung cancer and immunochemotherapy with *Propionibacterium granulosum* KP45. *Journal of Cancer Research and Clinical Oncology*, **109**, 72–7.

Rudge, P., Koetsier, J. C., Mertin, J., Beyer, J. O. M., van Walbeek, H. K., Jones, R. C. *et al.* (1989). Randomised double-blind controlled trial of cyclosporin in multiple sclerosis. *Journal of Neurology, Neurosurgery and Psychiatry*, **52**, 559–65.

Salo, O. and Lassus, A. (1983). Treatment of recurrent genital herpes with isoprinosine. *European Journal of Sexually Transmitted Diseases*, **1**, 101–5.

Sany, J., Clot, J., Bonneau, M., and Andary, M. (1982). Immunomodulating effect of human placenta-eluted gamma globulins in rheumatoid arthritis. *Arthritis and Rheumatism*, **25**, 17–24.

Savino, W., Dardenne, M., Marche, C., Trophilme, D., Dupuy, J-M., Pekovic, D. *et al.* (1986). Thymic epithelium in AIDS. An immunohistologic study. *American Journal of Pathology*, **122**, 302–7.

Scadding, G. K. and Brostoff, J. (1986). Low-dose sublingual therapy in patients with allergic rhinitis due to house dust mite. *Clinical Allergy*, **16**, 483–91.

Schiller, J. H., Storer, B., Dreicer, R., Rosenquist, D., Frontiera, M., and Carbone, P. P. (1989). Randomised phase II-III trial of combination beta and gamma interferons and etoposide and cisplatin in inoperable non-small cell cancer of the lung. *Journal of the National Cancer Institute*, **81**, 1739–43.

Schindler, J., Kennedy, S. M., and Wolfe, F. (1988). Potential of gamma-interferon in rheumatoid arthritis. *Advances in Inflammation Research*, **12**, 305–11.

Schonfeld, A., Nitke, S., Schattner, A., Wallach, D., Crespi, M., Hahn, T. *et al.* (1984). Intramuscular human interferon-beta injections in treatment of *condylomata acuminata*. *Lancet*, **i**, 1038–42.

Scott, G. M., Reed, S., Cartwright, T., and Tyrrell, D. (1980). Failure of human fibroblast interferon to protect against Rhinovirus infection. *Archives of Virology*, **65**, 135–9.

Scott, G. M., Phillpotts, R. J., Wallace, J., Gauci, C. L., Greiner, J., and Tyrrell, D. A. J. (1982). Prevention of rhinovirus colds by human Interferon alpha-2 from *Escherichia coli*. *Lancet*, **ii**, 186–9.

Sertoli, M. R., Guarneri, D., Rubagotti, A., Porcile, G., Nobile, M. T., and Rosso, R. (1987). Adjuvant immunochemotherapy in colorectal cancer Dukes C. *Oncology*, **44**, 78–81.

Silver, H. K. B., Connors, J. M., Kong, S., Karim, K. A., and Spinelli, J. J. (1988). Survival, response and immune effects in a prospectively randomised study of dose strategy for alpha-N1 interferon. *British Journal of Cancer*, **58**, 783–7.

Silvestris, F., Gernone, A., Frassanito, M. A., and Dammacco, F. (1989). Immunologic effects of long-term thymopentin treatment in patients with HIV-induced lymphadenopathy syndrome. *Journal of Laboratory and Clinical Medicine*, **113**, 139–44.

Smith, C. I. Kitchen, L. W., Scullard, G. H., Robinson, W. S., Gregory, P. B., and Merigan, T. C. (1982). Vidarabine monophosphate and human leukocyte Interferon in chronic hepatitis B infection. *Journal of the American Medical Association*, **247**, 2261–5.

Smith, P. G. (1988) Epidemiological methods to evaluate vaccine efficacy. *British Medical Bulletin*, **44**, 679–90.

Souter, R. G., Gill, P. G., Gunning, A. J., and Morris, P. J. (1981). Failure of specific active immunotherapy in lung cancer. *British Journal of Cancer*, **44**, 496–501.

Souter, R. G., Gill, P. G., and Morris, P. J. (1982). A trial of nonspecific immunotherapy using systemic *C. parvum* in treated patients with Dukes B and C colorectal cancer. *British Journal of Cancer*, **45**, 506–12.

Stanton, G. J., Weigent, D. A., Fleischmann, W. R., Dianzani, F., and Baron, S. (1987). Interferon review. *Investigative Radiology*, **22**, 259–73.

Steele, R. W., Myers, M. G., and Vincent, M. M. (1980). Transfer factor for the prevention of varicella-zoster infection in childhood leukemia. *New England Journal of Medicine*, **303**, 355–9.

Strander, H., Aparisi, T., Blomgren, H., Brostrom, L. A., Cantell, K., Einhorn, S. *et al.* (1982). Adjuvant interferon treatment of human osteosarcoma. *Recent Results in Cancer Research*, **80**, 103–7.

Szmuness, W., Stevens, C. E., Harley, E. J., Zang, E. A., Oleszko, W. R., William, D. C. *et al.* (1980). Hepatitis B vaccine: demonstration of efficacy in a controlled clinical trial in a high-risk population in the United States. *New England Journal of Medicine*, **303**, 833–41.

Szmuness, W., Stevens, C. E., Harley, E. J., Zang, E. A., Alter, H. J., Taylor, P. E. *et al.* (1982). Hepatitis B vaccine in medical staff of hemodialysis units. *New England Journal of Medicine*, **307**, 1481–6.

Talpaz, M., McCredie, K. B., Mavligit, G. M., and Gutterman, J. U. (1983). Leukocyte interferon-induced myeloid cytoreduction in chronic myelogenous leukaemia. *Blood*, **62**, 689–92.

Talpaz, M., Kantarjian, H. M., McCredie, K., Trujillo, J. M., Keating, M. J., and Gutterman, J. U. (1986). Hematologic remission and cytogenetic improvement induced by recombinant human interferon alpha$_A$ in chronic myelogenous leukaemia. *New England Journal of Medicine*, **314**, 1065–9.

Tan, E. G., Cohen, A. S., Fries, J. F., Masi, A. T., McShane, D. J., Rothfield, N. F. *et al.* (1982). The 1982 revised criteria for the classification of systemic lupus erythematosus. *Arthritis and Rheumatism*, **25**, 1271–7.

Tanphaichitra, D. and Srimuang, S. (1987). Efficacy of acyclovir combined with immunopotentiating agents in the treatment of varicella-zoster. *Journal of Antimicrobial Chemotherapy*, **19**, 255–62.

Thompson, A. J., Brady, J., Kidd, P., and Fefer, A. (1985). Recombinant alpha$_2$ interferon in the treatment of hairy cell leukaemia. *Cancer Treatment Reports*, **69**, 791–3.

Thompson, D. M. P., Major, P. P., Shuster, J., and Gold, P. (1988). Tumour immunology. In: *Immunological diseases* (eds M. Samter, D. W. Talmage, M. M. Frank, K. F. Austen, and H. N. Claman), vol. I, pp. 521–51. Little, Brown, Boston, USA.

Thompson, R. A., Bousquet, J., Cohen, S., Frei, P. C., Jager, L., Lambert, P. H. *et al.* (1989). The current status of allergen immunotherapy (hyposensitisation). Report of a WHO/IUIS working group. *Allergy*, **44**, 369–79.

Tindall, R. S. A., Rollins, J. A., Phillips, J. T., Greenlee, R. G.,Wells, L. and Belendiuk, G. (1987). Preliminary results of a double-blind, randomised, placebo-controlled trial of cyclosporine in myasthenia gravis. *New England Journal of Medicine*, **316**, 719–24.

Turner, M. W., Yalcin, I., Soothill, J. F., Price, J. F., Warner, J. O., Hey, E. N. *et al.* (1984). *In vitro* investigations in asthmatic children undergoing hyposensitisation with tyrosine-adsorbed *Dermatophagoides pteronyssinus* antigen. *Clinical Allergy*, **14**, 221–31.

Uchida, A. and Micksche, M. (1983). Intrapleural administration of OK432 in cancer patients: activation of NK cells and reduction of suppressor cells. *International Journal of Cancer*, **31**, 1–5.

Uchino, H., Yasunaga, K. and Akatsuka, J-I. (1984). A cooperative clinical trial of high-dose immunoglobulin therapy in 177 cases of idiopathic thrombocytopaenic purpura. *Thombosis and Haemostasis*, **51**, 182–5.

Umeda, T. and Niijima, T. (1986). Phase II study of alpha-interferon in renal cell carcinoma: summary of three collaborative trials. *Cancer*, **58**, 1231–5.

van Joost, T., Bos, J. D., Heule, F., and Meinardi, M. M. H. M. (1988). Low-dose cyclosporin A in severe psoriasis. A double-blind study. *British Journal of Dermatology*, **118**, 183–90.

Vannini, A., Cembrano, S., Assetto, V., and Giannitelli, A. (1986). interferon-beta treatment of herpes simplex keratitis. *Ophthalmologica (Basel)*, **192**, 6–10.

van Rijthoven, A. W. A. M., Dijkmans, B. A. C., The, H. S. G., Hermans, J., Montnor-Beckers, Z. L. M. B., Jacobs, P. C. J. *et al.* (1986). Cyclosporin treatment for rheumatoid arthritis: a placebo-controlled, double-blind, multicentre study. *Annals of the Rheumatic Diseases*, **45**, 726–31.

Vaughan, C. (1990). America considers offering 'untried remedies' to people with AIDS. *New Scientist*, **31st March**.

Vesikari, T., Isolauri, E., D'Hondt, E., Delem, A., Andre, F. E., and Zissis, G. (1984). Protection of infants against rotavirus diarrhoea by RIT 4237 attenuated bovine rotavirus strain vaccine. *Lancet*, **i**, 977–81.

Vesikari, T., Isolauri, E., Delem, A., D'Hondt, E., Andre, F. E., Beards, G. M. *et al.* (1985). Clinical efficacy of the RIT 4237 live attenuated bovine rotavirus vaccine in infants vaccinated before a rotavirus epidemic. *Journal of Paediatrics*, **107**, 189–94.

Veys, E. M., Mielants, H., Verbruggen, G., Dhondt, E., Goethals, L., Cheroutre, L. *et al.* (1981). Levamisole as basic treatment of rheumatoid arthritis: longterm evaluation. *Journal of Rheumatology*, **8**, 45–56.

Veys, E. M., Mielants, H., Verbruggen, G., Grosclaude, J-P., Meyer, W., Galazka, A. *et al.* (1988). Interferon gamma in rheumatoid arthritis—A double-blind study comparing human recombinant interferon gamma with placebo. *Journal of Rheumatology*, **15**, 570–4.

Vogler, W. R., Winton, E. F., Gordon, D. S., Raney, M. R., Go, B., and Meyer, L. (1984). A randomised comparison of postremission therapy in acute myelogenous leukaemia: a Southeastern Cancer Study Group Trial. *Blood*, **63**, 1039–45.

Vogl, S. E., Schoenfeld, D. A., Kaplan, B. H., Lerner, H. J., Horton, J., Creech, R. H. *et al.* (1982). Methotrexate alone or with regional sub-cutaneous *Corynebacterium parvum* in the treatment of recurrent and metastatic squamous cancer of the head and neck. *Cancer*, **50**, 2295–300.

von Wussow, P., Block, B., Hartmann, F., and Deicher, H. (1988). Intralesional interferon-alpha therapy in advanced malignant melanoma. *Cancer*, **61**, 1071–4.

Weimar, W., Heijtink, R. A., Ten Kate, F. J. P., Schalm, S. W., Masurel, N., Schellekens, H. *et al.* (1980). Double-blind study of leucocyte Interferon administration in chronic HBsAg-positive hepatitis. *Lancet*, **i**, 336–8.

Weinblatt, M. E., Coblyn, J. S., Fraser, P. A., Anderson, R. J., Spragg, J., Trentham, D. E. *et al.* (1987). Cyclosporin A treatment of refractory rheumatoid arthritis. *Arthritis and Rheumatism*, **30**, 11–17.

Whicher, J. T. and Dieppe, P. A. (1985). Acute phase proteins. *Clinics in Immunology Allergy*, **5**, 425–446.

Whitehead, J. (1983). *The design and analysis of sequential clinical trials*. Ellis Horwood Press, Chichester.

Winston, D. J., Pollard, R. B., Ho, W. G., Gallagher, J. G., Rasmussen, L. E., Huang, S. N-Y. *et al.* (1982). Cytomegalovirus immune plasma in bone-marrow transplant recipients. *Annals of Internal Medicine*, **97**, 11–18.

Wong, V. C. W., Ip, H. M. H., Reesink, H. W., Lelie, P. N., Reerink-Brongers, E. E., Yeung, C. Y. *et al.* (1984). Prevention of the HBsAg carrier state in newborn infants of mothers who are chronic carriers of HBsAg and HBeAg by administration of hepatitis-B vaccine and hepatitis-B immunoglobulin. *Lancet*, **i**, 921–6.

Woodruff, M. and Walbaum, P. (1983). A phase-II trial of *Corynebacterium parvum* as adjuvant to surgery in the treatment of operable lung cancer. *Cancer Immunology and Immunotherapy*, **16**, 114–6.

Worman, C. P., Catovsky, D., Bevan, P. C., Camba, L., Joyner, M., and Green, P. J. (1985). Interferon is effective in hairy cell leukaemia. *British Journal of Haematology*, **60**, 759–63.

Wunderlich, M., Schiessel, R., Rainer, H., Rauhs, R., Kovats, E., Schemper, M. *et al.* (1985). Effect of adjuvant chemo- or immunotherapy on the prognosis of colorectal cancer operated for cure. *British Journal of Surgery*, **72**, S107–10.

Yasumoto, K., Yaita, H., Ohta, M., Azuma, I., Nomoto, K., Inokuchi, K., and Yamamura, Y. (1985). Randomly controlled study of chemotherapy versus chemoimmunotherapy in postoperative lung cancer patients. *Cancer Research*, **45**, 1413–17.

Yocum, D. E., Klippel, J. H., Wilder, R. L., Gerber, N. L., Austin, H. A., Wahl, S. M. *et al.* (1988). Cyclosporin A in severe, treatment-refractory rheumatoid arthritis. *Annals of Internal Medicine*, **109**, 863–9.

Yoshida, S., Tanaka, R., Takai, N., and Ono, K. (1988). Local administration of autologous lymphokine-activated killer cells and recombinant interleukin-2 to patients with malignant brain tumours. *Cancer Research*, **48**, 5011–6.

Ziegler, E. J., McCutchan, J. A., Fierer, J., Glauser, M. P., Sadoff, J. C., Douglas, H. *et al.* (1982). Treatment of gram-negative bacteremia and shock with human antiserum to a mutant *Escherichia coli*. *New England Journal of Medicine*, **307**, 1225–30.

Index

N.B. References to trials on particular drugs or diseases should generally be sought through the appendices to chapters five to eight. Drugs and diseases are listed here if they have been discussed in the context of particular points of clinical trial methodology. Drugs are also listed here if their mechanism of action was discussed in the text.

Index